IMAGINE

not as much

ENDORSEMENTS

In September of 2015, I received some news which would change my life forever. I was diagnosed with diabetes. At that point, it almost felt like a death sentence because I just felt like I could not change what was necessary to improve my health. It was shortly after receiving the diagnosis that I was told about *Imagine Not as Much* I started the classes in October of that year. There, I found acceptance and people who were struggling with the same issues. The Whisnants were welcoming, kind, and warm-hearted. They were people who understood the struggle and really wanted to help. Through the material they shared and their own experiences, I began to see some change. I began losing weight and improving my A1C. I am currently a diet-controlled diabetic! Had it not been for *Imagine Not as Much,* I would still be on medication and quite possibly headed for insulin dependence. These principles, though not new, are infused by the Whisnants with faith and a positivity that I did not find anywhere else! I owe them more than I can repay. They and their labor of love have been a great blessing to me.

—Douglas Risley

Imagine Not as Much has so many good ideas for losing weight and studying God's Word. One of my favorite things was the challenge that Nathan gave us each week. It helped me to stay on track with Bible study and losing weight.

—Diane E.

With *Imagine Not as Much,* I enjoyed including healthy snacks with Bible study and exercise.

—Brandy L.

My husband and I were blessed to be a part of the *Imagine Not as Much* class. Dr. Nathan and Ms. Tammy Whisnant developed—an informative, Christ-centered, and supportive program that has had very positive results not only for our congregation, but for our community as well. In an easy-to-understand method, Dr. Nathan and Tammy teach how to determine caloric needs, nutritional information of foods, and kinds of exercise by using examples and Scripture-based devotionals for inspiration and encouragement. The *Imagine Not as Much* class and book are focused on meeting the holistic needs of individuals and improving our health to honor God with our bodies. It was so encouraging to be a part of such a supportive class. By incorporating both physical and spiritual aspects, I not only lost weight but grew in my faith as well. Dr. Nathan and Tammy have truly heeded God's calling to minister to others with this program.

—Janet D. Ziegler
MsN, ACNP-BC

Very motivating program. Loved implementing Bible study and diet with exercise in *Imagine Not as Much.*

—Mitzi F.

I found the program easy to follow, and it worked. Watching calories and exercising works. It's just that simple with *Imagine Not as Much.*

—Lori B.

Imagine Not as Much is a relatable program from day one. Nathan and Tammy begin with testimonials of why they developed the program and how it has continued to affect their health and ministry. All of the common-sense information for healthy eating and exercise are included; plus, daily devotionals, challenges, and focus points keep one on track physically and spiritually. "Nathan's Notions" and "Tammy's Tidbits" give a sense of their personal commitment in my success with the program.

—Janet S.

Imagine Not as Much has helped me with meal planning. I like it because there are no "special" foods to prepare. My family can also enjoy eating, and it won't break the budget.

—Michelle Woodard

I have found *Imagine Not as Much* to be a great way to lose weight and strengthen your Christian faith at the same time. *Imagine Not as Much* teaches in a way that is no pressure. You are taught to be okay, even if you have setbacks. This book is a one-of-a-kind, and I wholeheartedly believe in it.

—Chris Reynolds

Imagine Not as Much is not a diet plan but a way of life. It teaches you ways to think about what you are eating. Eat what you like, but maybe not as much.

—Ann Reynolds

Imagine Not as Much is a Christ-centered eating plan to help you get to your goal for weight management. Researched well and presented in an easy-to-follow format, this program provides an exercise plan to fit in your lifestyle and daily devotions to keep you encouraged and motivated. Never embarrassment, only helpful advice and sharing. What's not to like? I have found that the only thing keeping you from success is yourself.

—Pam Stone

Imagine Not as Much has helped me in weight loss—sixteen pounds in thirteen weeks. This has been a lifestyle change in eating habits. I highly recommend it for people who want to improve health; it's not just about weight loss, but nutritionally and spiritually based as well. This has helped my health in:

      Reduced cholesterol: 210—175

      Lower blood pressure: 135/90—110/72

      Lower blood sugar: 155—90

      Lower triglycerides: 450—155

—David Powers

Imagine Not as Much has been a lifesaver for me. I had gained an excess of thirty pounds, and going through this class has helped me to lose twenty-one of that! Nathan and Tammy are a great inspiration. They are true examples of what a faith-based weight loss program is all about. Any questions or concerns you have, they both lovingly answer. They are always helpful and caring; no matter if you lose every week or you gain, they never judge. This is my second time taking the class, and I recommend it to everyone. It is truly a lifestyle change for the better!

—Dana Powers

Although we started *Imagine Not as Much* on week three, following my doctor's recommendation to this program, we felt very welcome. We were inspired by the passages from Scripture chosen to begin each chapter. The suggestions/tips we've received from the other participants are very much appreciated. We have tried them all. We admire the non-judgmental and kindness approach. Also, the positive reinforcement is outstanding. We can also relate to all the personal testimonies. We are looking forward to trying all the recipes. They sound yummy! I (Maria) have tweaked my diet over many years and have been able to lose sixty-one pounds on my own. But I reached a plateau and hope these further changes to my diet will help me to lose more. The best part is that my husband (Jerome) has agreed wholeheartedly to do this with me. So, yes, thank you for this excellent program.

—Maria and Jerome Dixon

IMAGINE

not as much

13 Weeks to Better Spiritual and Physical Health

NATHAN AND TAMMY WHISNANT

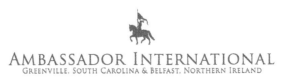

AMBASSADOR INTERNATIONAL
GREENVILLE, SOUTH CAROLINA & BELFAST, NORTHERN IRELAND

www.ambassador-international.com

Imagine Not As Much

13 Weeks to Better Spiritual and Physical Health
©2020 by Nathan and Tammy Whisnant

ISBN: 978-1-62020-910-3
eISBN: 978-1-62020-923-3

Cover Design and Page Layout by Hannah Nichols
eBook Conversion by Anna Riebe Raats

Neither the publisher nor the author is engaged in rendering professional advice or services to the individual reader. The ideas, procedures, and suggestions contained in this book are not intended as a substitute for consulting with your physician. All matters regarding your health require medical supervision. Neither the author nor the publisher shall be liable or responsible for any loss or damage allegedly arising from any information or suggestion in this book.

Unless otherwise noted, all Scripture quotations are taken from the Christian Standard Bible®, Copyright © 2017 by Holman Bible Publishers. Used by permission. Christian Standard Bible® and CSB® are federally registered trademarks of Holman Bible Publishers.

AMBASSADOR INTERNATIONAL
Emerald House
411 University Ridge, Suite B14
Greenville, SC 29601, USA
www.ambassador-international.com

AMBASSADOR BOOKS
The Mount
2 Woodstock Link
Belfast, BT6 8DD, Northern Ireland, UK
www.ambassadormedia.co.uk

The colophon is a trademark of Ambassador, a Christian publishing company.

We dedicate this book first and foremost to our Lord and Savior Jesus Christ, Who has done above and beyond what we could ever have asked or thought.

We dedicate this book to our daughters, Cassie Edinger and Cara Roberson, and our grandchildren: Angel, Preston, James, Adri, Madeline, and Duke. You are the source of our imagination!

We dedicate this book to our parents, Marvin and Ruth Whisnant and Richard and Martha Hester, for instilling in us faith, hard work, and perseverance.

"Now to him who is able to do above and beyond all that we ask or think according to the power that works in us—to him be glory" (Eph. 3:20-21a).

CONTENTS

ACKNOWLEDGMENTS

A lot of people have made this book possible. We want to thank just a few of the many:

Airline Baptist Church for giving Nathan the time and opportunity to write and teach *Imagine Not as Much*! They have truly offered help and support through prayer, encouragement, comprising the first group of Imaginators, and providing copies of the book for free to those who took the class at the church.

Nathan's brother, Mitchell Whisnant, for his comments that spurred us to write this book. He said early in 2015, "Nathan, you need to write down what you did to lose weight, so you can help others. People may not attend church to hear you preach, but they will attend to lose weight!"

Tammy's sister and mother, Julie and Martha Hester, for listening to the incessant rewrites.

Our two daughters, Cassie Edinger and Cara Roberson, and their families, who have listened, given advice, and even groaned at times at our ideas. Thank you for your honest input. "Just imaginate, girls!"

Michael and Betty Whisnant, Vicki Whisnant (Mitchell's wife), Trish and Jimmy Delano, Helen and Gene Hall, Carrie and Mark Gustafson, and Peggy and Richie Nix for being the best supportive siblings we could ever have.

Our families for understanding when we missed valuable family time.

Dr. Bill Patterson, our mentor who has not only guided us through the writing, editing, and publishing process, but who also has given inspirational advice. He and his late wife, Debbie, have acted as our biggest cheerleaders in the surrounding community. Bill, we value your expertise and consider your friendship a treasure.

Our graphic designer and niece, Kathleen Stanley, for an artistic eye to bring to life the first cover of the original manuscript of *Imagine Not as Much!* and our current Imagine Ministries brand.

Airline Baptist Church's former secretary, Kathleen Daly, for the countless hours of copying and assembling the original manuscript, along with the many unpublished rewrites.

Our photographer, Carolyn Allen, for making the photo shoot pleasant and painless.

HSC Medical Billing and parent company Harding, Shymanski & Company, for jumpstarting Tammy's weight loss journey by providing an on-site weight loss class at half the cost.

Ambassador International and Sam Lowry, for helping us get our message of Christ-centered weight loss to more people than we could ever imagine.

Last, but not least, our Imaginators, who have successfully completed at least one cycle of Imagine Not as Much, lost weight, and kept it off. Your critique, ideas for improvement, and patience as each cycle changed have proved invaluable. We love you guys, and you will always hold a special place in our hearts. Forgive us for not naming all of you. But know that our success is your success.

FOREWORD
BY DR. BILL PATTERSON

Nathan and Tammy Whisnant have written a wonderful book on weight loss, based on biblical teachings. Serious Christians who seriously want to get in shape will want to read this book.

I took the Imagine Not as Much course taught by the Whisnants and lost eight pounds over twelve weeks. I took it again and lost five more pounds. The amazing thing? I wasn't hungry. The Whisnants taught me how to lose the weight while eating what I wanted. Since completing the second course a year-and-a-half ago, I have lost an additional nineteen pounds and am now at my target weight. Unlike many weight-loss programs, theirs teaches how to keep off the lost poundage.

The Whisnants combined up-to-date coaching on weight loss with biblical teachings of yielding to the Lord Jesus and viewing our bodies as the temples of the Holy Spirit. They also modeled what they taught by showing how they lost weight and how we can lose, too.

Over the last several years, the Whisnants have taught Imagine Not as Much in more than ten settings. Each time, remarkable stories emerge of people whose doctors advised them to eliminate or reduce their medications due to their having lost weight and having developed better fitness. Others recall feeling resigned to being overweight the rest of their lives, only to apply the principles in this book and then getting their lives and their weight under control again. Nathan recently called me with news that a local doctor, having seen the results of Imagine Not as Much in several patients, has begun referring patients to the program!

Wonderful encouragers, the Whisnants will guide you in doing what they have seen dozens and dozens of others do—begin to view life in a spiritual way in which eating is enjoyed but placed under the control of the Master. You will find, as I did, that you enjoy the tastes of food even more when in its proper place in your life.

If consuming too much—or too much of the wrong things—is a problem for you, invest in this book. Put its principles into practice. Yield yourself more fully to the Lord. See food take its proper role in your life. Watch your body begin to shape up. Relish life more. Enjoy letting Jesus be Lord of your carbs and your meats, of your cardio and your metabolism. Let Him be Lord of your drinks and desserts and desires. Feast on Him. The Whisnants will show you how in this delightful book. You'll be glad you did!

PREFACE

Thank you for choosing *Imagine Not as Much*. We wrote this book out of a desire to help those who have lost hope in their weight-loss journey and/or for those who want to begin the journey. We hope that this book will help you to lose weight and grow in your relationship with the Lord. We do not think of this as a diet but as a journey, one that we want to empower you to travel throughout your lifetime. As you put into practice what you read, we expect that you will experience effective, permanent weight-loss, lowered A1C, lowered blood pressure, and lowered cholesterol. We also anticipate you will discover the confidence that you can do this for the rest of your life.

We wrote this book with leading groups in mind, but you can embark on this journey on your own. We do encourage you to find a local group or start an Imagine Not as Much support group in your church or community.

Between us, we have lost almost a hundred pounds. We both know the challenges that people face on a weight-loss journey and have addressed them in the book. We will spend three chapters on each of the following four fitness aspects: nutritional, physical, motivational, and spiritual. In nutritional fitness, we will talk about setting goals, setting your calorie intake, what types of food to eat, and when and how to eat. In physical fitness, we will talk about the different types of activity and choosing the ones best for you. In motivational fitness, we will talk about setting your mind to this lifestyle change and conquering roadblocks that you may face. In spiritual fitness, we will talk about beginning your relationship with Jesus and ways to deepen that relationship. We have also included a thirteen-week devotional that includes all four fitness aspects, in addition to the benefits of water, time management, and friends.

Imagine getting up from the dinner table satisfied, yet not stuffed. Imagine having the energy and desire to take a walk in the park or a run on the beach. Imagine the wonderful, horrible feeling of your clothes no longer fitting because of your smaller waist size. Imagine having a sweeter relationship with the Lord with a healthier body. All of these things have already happened to many who have read our book, and we expect them to happen to you as you *Imagine Not as Much*!

FIRST FOCUS: NUTRITIONAL FITNESS

"So, whether you eat or drink, or whatever you do, do everything for the glory of God" (1 Cor. 10:31).

WEEK 1: GOALS

The material that comprises this training includes our personal stories, what worked for us in each of the four fitness areas, and how we plan on helping you reach your weight-loss goal.

In the next thirteen weeks, you can expect support, encouragement, accountability, fellowship, new knowledge, and purpose in a safe group environment. We have learned that people in a group lose more weight than those who try it alone, especially if they stay with the group for the entire thirteen weeks.

We have not reinvented the wheel. Common knowledge tells us that to lose weight, we must eat less and exercise more. In *Imagine Not as Much*, we can help you know how to do those two things easily and practically for your current lifestyle or challenges. We suggest you consult with your doctor before engaging in any new physical activity. If you do not belong to an Imagine Not as Much group, think about starting one!

We have included lessons on four fitness areas needed to effectively lose weight: nutritional fitness, physical fitness, motivational fitness, and spiritual fitness. We have also provided a daily devotional reading following each week. Each week of devotions contains seven foci: the four previous fitness areas and the benefits of water, effective time management, and friends. We have included "Nathan's Notions" and "Tammy's Tidbits" for each day. We trust these will help you keep your focus of losing weight as a way to give glory to God. We wrote *Imagine Not as Much* as a Christ-centered strategy to help you reach your goals.

NATHAN'S STORY

Once I decided to lose weight, I would do okay for a while and then gain back everything I had lost. A couple things happened in a short period of time that convinced me I had to change. I noticed while tying my shoes, I got out of breath, and my face turned red because my belly pressed on my knees as I bent over. I also noticed that whenever one of my grandkids asked me to play, I would most often respond with, "Not right now. Papaw just does not feel up to it." After a while, they quit asking. I realized then that if I did not change my ways, I would shorten my time of ministry either because of incapacitation or early death due to complications from obesity.

In May of 2013, I decided to do something about it. I wanted that something to last for a lifetime, not just a short duration. I weighed 215 pounds. I set a goal to lose thirty pounds in thirty weeks. I made it in twenty-six weeks, reaching my weight loss goal on November 4, 2013.

I have maintained my weight ever since. Currently, I weigh 180, give or take a couple of pounds. I have weighed as little as 175 pounds and as heavy as 190 pounds since I reached my goal. I know how to gain a few when needed, and I know how to lose a few when needed.

TAMMY'S STORY

My desire to lose weight began after Nathan lost his weight. He had more energy than I had, and he looked so skinny! He never said anything to me about my weight but always showed support. I also wanted to feel better. At one time, I took two blood pressure medications and medicine for high cholesterol. And quite honestly, I began to feel convicted about my sin of overeating. I felt I had compromised my testimony because one could tell by looking at me that I overate on a daily basis. I lost fifty pounds with another weight-loss program, then switched to Imagine Not as Much for the final ten pounds. I lost weight, and now I feel marvelous!

YOUR STORY

We want to share with you what we have learned and how to apply it specifically to your lives. We want to help you reach your goal. Why do you want to lose weight?

_____

_____

_____

_____

Now, how did we do it?

Let's start with nutritional fitness.

We used the Food Guide Pyramid (U.S. Department of Agriculture) to direct our nutritional intake for each day. We decided our weight loss goal by referring to a BMI (body mass index) chart. Nathan came up with the goal of twenty-four BMI, or 185 pounds.

Next, we determined how much we could eat and still lose weight. Nathan learned if he ate ten times his target weight for calorie intake, he would lose weight. So, he came up with an eating plan of 1,850 calories a day. We learned that to lose weight, we needed to eat five or six times a day: three meals and two to three snacks.

Now, let's work on your goals.

Let's start with your weight loss goal. You may refer to a BMI chart on your smartphone for help determining a healthy weight for you.

RECORD YOUR CURRENT WEIGHT   NATHAN'S EXAMPLE

_____   215 pounds

Record your weight loss goal

_____   185 pounds

Subtract your ideal weight from your current weight, and record the total number of pounds you want to lose for a healthy weight.

Nathan's example

_____   215

                                                            -185
                                              _____

                                                             30

To determine your calorie intake, multiply your target weight by ten. Record that number below. This number must not dip below 1200 calories.

_____   185 X 10 = 1,850

For the next thirteen weeks, set a goal for the number of pounds you want to lose. A person can achieve healthy weight loss by losing one to two pounds a week, meaning between thirteen and twenty-six pounds. Record your short-term goal below.

_____   13 pounds

We have provided Nathan's example of how he planned his nutritional intake to reach his goal of 185 pounds by eating 1,850 calories a day. He consumed three meals a day at approximately five hundred calories each and three snacks a day around one hundred calories each, with fifty fun calories to do with whatever he wanted!

Nathan's example

Target Weight	185	
Multiply weight by 10	1850	equals daily caloric intake
Number of snacks X 100	300	
Subtract snacks number		
from daily caloric intake	1550	equals total meal calories
Divide total meal calories by 3	500	(516.66) equals each meal value

Record above information below:

Breakfast	500
Snack	100
Lunch	500
Snack	100
Dinner	500
Snack	100
Buffer	50
Total Daily Calories	1850

Your Information

Target Weight   _____

Multiply target weight by 10   _____ equals daily caloric intake

Number of snacks X 100   _____

Subtract snacks number

from daily caloric intake   _____ equals total meal calories

Divide total meal calories by 3   _____ equals each meal value

Record above information below:

Breakfast	_____
Snack	_____
Lunch	_____
Snack	_____
Dinner	_____
Snack	_____
Buffer	_____
Total Daily Calories	_____

In the next chapter, we will discuss healthy food choices.

WEEK 1: DAY 1

Memory Verse: "So, whether you eat or drink, or whatever you do, do everything for the glory of God" (1 Cor. 10:31).

Challenge: This week, track the calories you eat each day in comparison to the calories you need to eat to lose weight.

Focus: Nutritional Fitness

NATHAN'S NOTIONS

Our memory verse reminds us that we should eat for God's glory. I did not think much of what I ate as it related to my walk with Christ; nor did I deal with my sin of gluttony, thinking, "Who does it hurt?" Well, it hurts God. He has designed our bodies in a way that when we follow Him in obedience, everything works perfectly. On the opposite side, when we abuse our bodies by filling it with junk, things begin to act out of kilter. I repented of my sin of gluttony, determined how many daily calories my body needed, and aligned my calories to the proper amount for my height. Now when I eat or drink, I ask myself, "Does this bring glory to God?"

Let's define God's glory. The Greek word for glory, *doxan,* translates to the English word *doxology,* meaning, "praise to God."[1] God's glory entails anything and everything that we do that praises God. We will unpack understanding God's glory today and tomorrow.

God's glory begins in the life of someone who has a personal relationship with Jesus. You cannot praise God if you reject His Son as Savior. Being a moral person but not having a relationship with Jesus works the same as mixing poison with good food: you end up with a poisoned mess. A parallel passage to our memory verse clearly identifies Jesus Christ as the only Way to do everything for God's glory. It reads, "And whatever you do, in word or in deed, do everything in the name of the Lord Jesus, giving thanks to God the Father through him" (Col. 3:17).

God's glory displays direct service to God. We serve God for His glory when we worship Him with a sincere heart, engage in Christian labor, and faithfully serve Him. Today, choose to do everything for God's glory by praising Him in what you eat and drink.

---

1 Gerhard Kittel, "The NT Use of *doxa,*" *Theological Dictionary of the New Testament* (Grand Rapids: Wm. B. Eerdmans Publishing Company, 1964), 2:237-251.

TAMMY'S TIDBITS

Begin today recording everything you eat in a food journal. Try this for the entire week. This will help you pinpoint challenges. You might discover you eat more than you think. You might also find when and how you can replace unhealthy choices for healthy ones. Recording your nutritional activity in a journal will help you track your progress in the *Imagine Not as Much* journey.

WEEK 1: DAY 2

Memory Verse: "So, whether you eat or drink, or whatever you do, do everything for the glory of God" (1 Cor. 10:31).

Challenge: This week, track the calories each day you eat in comparison to the calories you need to eat to lose weight.

Focus: Benefits of Water

NATHAN'S NOTIONS

Our memory verse this week reminds us that what we drink should bring God glory. I used to drink three or four sugary, citrus-flavored soft drinks each day and sweet tea with two meals a day without giving it a second thought. I found out that God designed us to drink water as the best thing to bring Him glory. I also found out that many times, we confuse thirst with hunger.[2] Drinking water may prevent us from eating unnecessarily and provide our bodies with what it truly thirsts: refreshment with pure, wonderful water.

Yesterday, we focused on our personal relationship with God and serving Him. Another thing to understand in doing everything for God's glory embodies duty to ourselves. God has created us, and thus, we need to treat the body He has created with respect. We should try to improve ourselves each day; to grow in grace each day; and to increase in nutritional, physical, motivational, and spiritual fitness each day. We should never reach satisfaction in our journey toward fitness, but find ways to improve, even with something small.

Additionally, God's glory embraces duty to others. If we truly want to praise God with everything we do, we must treat every person He has created as special. We treat others for God's glory by loving them as we love ourselves, by trying not to offend their consciences, by trying not to hinder their spiritual life through causing them to sin, by practicing self-denial for their benefit, and by earnestly seeking their salvation.

TAMMY'S TIDBITS

This week, replace one of your normal drinks with water. Instead of a diet drink or tea, drink water with one meal. If you continue with this habit, it won't take long to discover that you enjoy the taste of pure, clean water!

---

2 David Zinczenko and Matt Goudling, *Eat This Not That! Restaurant Guide: The No-Diet Weight Loss Solution* (New York: Rodale, 2010), 13.

WEEK 1: DAY 3

Memory Verse: "So, whether you eat or drink, or whatever you do, do everything for the glory of God" (1 Cor. 10:31).

Challenge: This week, track the calories each day you eat in comparison to the calories you need to eat to lose weight.

Focus: Physical Fitness

NATHAN'S NOTIONS

"Whatever you do." Certainly, this phrase encompasses what we do with our bodies on a regular basis. As an overweight person, I rationalized not participating in physical fitness. I did not make the connection that physical fitness might actually help me feel better. I did not want to give my daily bodily activities to God's glory. Once the Lord convicted me, I quickly learned that what I did or did not do with my body reflected my desire to do everything for God's glory.

How do we carry out that desire? Simply fall in line with God's purposes. God wants everyone to experience eternal life through a personal relationship with Jesus. Can what I eat and drink bring God glory? Yes, if it helps someone come to know Jesus. I needed to take seriously my addiction to food, my sin of gluttony, and how all that related to someone not accepting Jesus. Now, I live each day with God's purposes in mind.

Another way is to revere God's laws. As a people of grace, the Old Testament laws do not constrain us, but can show the seriousness of our commitment to God's glory.

In addition, we should utter God's praises with every breath we take. We can do this by conditioning our bodies physically, so we can do as much as possible to serve Him. When people see us, they should see our commitment about how our bodies utter praise to God. We should do everything for God's glory!

TAMMY'S TIDBITS

Today, enjoy nature by taking a walk giving God praise, glory, and honor!

WEEK 1: DAY 4

Memory Verse: "So, whether you eat or drink, or whatever you do, do everything for the glory of God" (1 Cor. 10:31).

Challenge: This week, track the calories each day you eat in comparison to the calories you need to eat to lose weight.

Challenge Check-up: What surprised you as you compared what you ate to what you should eat?

Focus: Benefits of Effective Time Management

NATHAN'S NOTIONS

When we use our time for God's glory, it allows us to take control of our lives instead of losing control to outside forces. It also allows us to spend our time effectively serving Him, instead of thinking about when we will eat again or how to work in a junk food fix!

We suffer serious consequences when we do not do everything for God's glory—such as confusion, contradiction, and chaos. Confusion and contradiction occur when we say one thing, but our actions say another. For instance, we claim Jesus as Lord, yet it remains painfully clear that we have not yielded to Jesus the control over our appetites and our activities. We preach with our actions the Lordship of Jesus over the spiritual things in our lives but not the secular. In the writings of Paul and everywhere else in Scripture, you will never find a disconnect between the sacred and the secular or a divide between the religious and the regular activities of life. Everything becomes sacred when we belong to the Lord, including what we eat, what we drink, and how we spend our time.

Chaos occurs in our lives when we refuse to give God our time. When we do everything for God's glory, including giving Him our entire day, we will find the peace that goes beyond understanding as we devote ourselves to Him. When we waste our time, we rob God, injure others, and realize little profit from our efforts. Effective time management conveys giving your daily activities to the glory of God! Today, take control over your life by giving God your calendar. You will never regret it.

TAMMY'S TIDBITS

Planning meals has proved to be an effective time management tool. You will know ahead of time what you will eat, so you can buy the right foods and prepare the right portions, taking the guess work out of healthy eating.

WEEK 1: DAY 5

Memory Verse: "So, whether you eat or drink, or whatever you do, do everything for the glory of God" (1 Cor. 10:31).

Challenge: This week, track the calories you eat each day in comparison to the calories you need to eat to lose weight.

Focus: Motivational Fitness

NATHAN'S NOTIONS

We can experience several benefits when we begin to do everything for God's glory. Each one of these will help us develop motivational fitness by keeping our minds focused. Doing everything for God's glory delivers us from the miserable existence of self-seeking, self-centered actions. Selfishness causes moods to change radically in a short period of time; good things create happiness, and bad things manifest sadness or anger. Doing everything for God's glory releases us from the moody yo-yo and helps us to focus on discovering His work in our midst. It delivers us from the murky atmosphere of an earthly-focused existence into the beautiful and serene atmosphere of a heavenly-minded existence. We begin to focus on eternal values and significance and how this affects the people around us. We no longer run the rat race. Rather, we have a keen sense of serving God in whatever task we find at hand.

Not only does it help our motivational fitness to do everything for God's glory, but it also benefits society. We begin to ask ourselves, "How will what I do help someone else?" The more people dedicate themselves to serving God, the better society will become. It satisfies our deep need to do something important and significant. When we successfully keep God's glory as our focus, we will never need to feel ashamed. And we can practice this for eternity. The ones who have gone on and the angels in Heaven currently do everything for God's glory. Once we leave this earth and join them, we will participate in the same joyous activity!

TAMMY'S TIDBITS

Losing weight begins with a change of mind. Decide today that you will eat healthy and exercise. Take personal responsibility.

WEEK 1: DAY 6

Memory Verse: "So, whether you eat or drink, or whatever you do, do everything for the glory of God" (1 Cor. 10:31).

Challenge: This week, track the calories you eat each day in comparison to the calories you need to eat to lose weight.

Focus: Benefits of Friends

NATHAN'S NOTIONS

I want to focus on one word from our memory verse—*panta,* translated as "everything."[3] *Panta* describes absolutely everything to the smallest minutia with nothing left out. *Panta* holds special significance to us as we look at the benefits of friends. Even our choice of friends and what we decide to do with them should give God glory. When alone, we sometimes eat right, exercise regularly, and get plenty of sleep; but we have some friends that will derail our efforts of living to the glory of God. They may not mean to be negative or have an awareness of their negative impact on our efforts. Hence, the importance of a couple of things.

We must let our current friends know that we have embarked on a lifestyle change. The things that we once did without thinking about, we have to stop. Our current friends need to know that something has changed inside of us and about the sincerity of our commitment to do everything for God's glory. At the same time, we must surround ourselves with friends on the same weight-loss journey. Imagine Not as Much classes combine our help with people in the group to assist you in reaching your weight-loss goal. The friends you meet in class will encourage you to operate with transparency, helping you to remain honest with yourself and your journey's progress. The class can pray for your struggles, celebrate your victories, and help you through plateaus.

TAMMY'S TIDBITS

Nathan and I would strongly encourage you to attend the Imagine Not as Much classes weekly. We have seen evidence that participating in a group setting leads to more effective weight loss. It's not too late to invite a friend to join you next week.

---

3 Joseph Henry Thayer, *A Greek-English Lexicon of the New Testament* (Edinburgh: T & T Clark, 1901), 476.

WEEK 1: DAY 7

Memory Verse: "So, whether you eat or drink, or whatever you do, do everything for the glory of God" (1 Cor. 10:31).

Challenge: This week, track the calories you eat each day in comparison to the calories you need to eat to lose weight.

Challenge Carryover: As you carry over this weekly challenge into life, exercise awareness of the calories you eat each day to stay on track. You don't have to count them strictly; just have a general ballpark figure in mind.

Focus: Spiritual Fitness

NATHAN'S NOTIONS

We have looked at many things about doing everything for God's glory. God's divine presence exists in everything He has created. We cannot escape God's presence in our everyday lives. Instead of ignoring Him or running from Him, our natural response should bring Him glory.

God has absolute sovereignty over everything He has created. "For from him and through him and to him are all things. To him be the glory forever. Amen" (Rom. 11:36). His absolute sovereignty also shows clearly in our personal redemption. When we invite Jesus into our hearts as Lord, we become children of God. We belong to God. Since we belong to God, He reigns over our actions.

Doing everything for God's glory transforms a monotonous string of trivialities into an amazing string of events that really matter: giving God glory in everything we eat, everything we drink, and everything else we do.

And most importantly, God told us to bring Him glory! Greek syntax (the order of words in a sentence) will often move words around based upon emphasis. If a word appears at the beginning or end of a sentence out of order, it signifies something important. In our memory verse, *poieite,* translated as "do," ends the verse.[4] The last few words of 1 Corinthians 10:31 literally read, "all things to the glory of God, do." God says do not take this "do" as a mere suggestion. Do not just ponder on it. "This thing of giving Me glory," God says, "do!" Do not consider it for a period of time before action; do it. "So, whether you eat or drink, or whatever you do, do everything for the glory of God." Do it because God said so!

---

4 Jay P. Green, Sr., ed., *The Interlinear Hebrew/Greek-English Bible* (Lafayette: Associated Publishers & Authors, Inc., 1976-1984), 4:468.

TAMMY'S TIDBITS

Continue with your daily devotion. It will encourage you in this weight-loss journey. Planning your devotion time stands in equal importance as planning your meals and physical activity.

FIRST FOCUS: NUTRITIONAL FITNESS

"Now to him who is able to do above and beyond all that we ask or think according to the power that works in us—to him be glory" (Eph. 3:20-21a).

WEEK 2: MEAL AND SNACK PLANNING

In Nathan's research, he learned that the *kind* of calories carried just as much importance as the *number* of calories in achieving weight loss. He needed to find the greatest benefit from the calories he consumed.

He chose primarily whole wheat starches, fresh or frozen vegetables and fruits, fat-free dairy, and lean meat. And the good stuff had to taste really, really good to satisfy him in small portions. He utilized six sections of the Food Guide Pyramid for guidance. You can follow his example.

The Pyramid recommends six to eleven servings of bread, cereal, rice, and pasta per day. Choose whole grain bread instead of white, cereals that have a high fiber content, brown or wild rice instead of white, and whole wheat pastas.

Two to four servings per day in the vegetable group are also recommended. Choose fresh or frozen over canned, and experiment with those not familiar to you. Try grilling or roasting your vegetables with a small amount of olive oil and adding seasonings you enjoy.

The fruit group in the Pyramid suggests two to four servings per day. Choose fresh or frozen over canned, but if canned, choose light or sugar-free. Experiment with new kinds of fruit.

In the milk, yogurt, and cheese group, two to three servings per day is the recommendation. Choose low-fat or fat-free options. Women over the age of fifty require at least three servings of dairy a day.

The meat, poultry, fish, dry beans, eggs, and nuts group should include two to three servings per day. Choose lean cuts of meat and wild fish over farm-raised fish.

Use the fats, oils, and sweets group sparsely. When cooking, choose extra virgin olive oil, and try to have no more than two servings per day from this group.

To have an idea of the size of suggested servings, refer to Appendix B at the end of the book for examples from each food group.

Let's start with the snacks. Nathan wanted them to contain approximately one hundred calories each for a total of three hundred calories at the end of the day. He loves chocolate, so he had to incorporate that as part of the equation. He likes repetition, so he knew he did not need a lot, just a few that he could rotate. Oh, and one more thing—for them to work for

Nathan, the morning and afternoon snacks had to fit on his person throughout the day. He typically wears a shirt and tie with a sport coat and matching pants. He wanted to choose snacks that would easily fit into his pockets.

He came up with the following snacks for the morning and afternoon: fudge-covered pretzels (100-calorie package), pastry crisps (100 calories), two triple berry fruit chewy cookies (100 calories), a box of raisins (90 calories), fifteen almonds (80 calories), a granola bar (100 calories), and fruit & grain bars (130 calories). For the evening snacks he chose some type of low-calorie ice cream (100-120 calories), and chocolate-covered granola bars (140 calories).

Nathan learned a basic principle of nutritional fitness:

CHOOSE ONLY FOODS YOU ENJOY!

What a simple yet powerful revelation for him. Diets did not work for him because he forced himself to eat things he did not like, thinking the end justified the means. He did not really enjoy the food he ate; he just wanted to lose weight. Once he learned that he could actually eat the foods he enjoyed and lose weight at the same time, his whole attitude changed.

Next, Nathan needed to determine what he would eat for breakfast. Keeping the Food Guide Pyramid in mind, along with healthy choices, he came up with four that he enjoys. They each contain approximately five hundred calories. They include two toaster pastries with one cup of 1% milk and coffee; two cups of wheat and rice flakes with raisins and oat clusters cereal, one cup of 1% milk, 1 Tbsp. flax-seed, and coffee; two waffles, ¼ cup of regular syrup, one cup of 1% milk, butter spray, and coffee; and half a cup of regular oatmeal, one cup of 1% milk, 1 Tbsp. flax-seed, two slices of whole wheat toast, butter spray, 2 Tbsp. regular jelly, and coffee.

After the breakfasts, Nathan had to find some simple yet healthy lunches that he could eat on a regular basis and enjoy. He came up with the two sandwiches made with four slices of whole wheat bread, two slices of fat-free cheese, and one package of sliced honey roasted turkey, sixteen reduced-fat chips, with regular whipped salad dressing and mustard on the sandwiches; one can of chunky sirloin burger soup with two slices of whole wheat bread containing one teaspoon of margarine on each slice; chicken-based frozen steamer bowl with two slices of whole wheat bread containing one teaspoon of margarine on each slice; and four cups of spring mix lettuce, one 8 oz. package of cooked chicken, one tomato, ¼ cup of dried cranberries, 2 Tbsp. fat-free dressing, and ¼ cup of Colby Jack shredded cheese.

For breakfast, Tammy typically eats toast (one thinly sliced whole grain bread) with butter spray, a bowl of fruit (½ a cup frozen mango and ½ a cup of frozen cherries sweetened with artificial sweetener), and one cup of skim milk. She also has a cup of black coffee with artificial sweetener. Sometimes, she will have low-fat, maple, brown sugar oatmeal with one cup of skim milk.

For lunch, she has one ounce of turkey on one thinly sliced whole grain bread. She also adds lettuce, tomato, and mustard to the sandwich. Celery cut up into bite-size pieces add crunch; she eats that instead of chips.

Snacks consist of twelve grapes with one low-fat string cheese; one eighty-calorie Greek nonfat flavored yogurt with any kind of fruit; one cup of fat-free cottage cheese with tomato or peaches in light syrup with the syrup drained; hummus with red, yellow, or green peppers; or ninety-calories baked brownie bars. Tammy tries to have three servings of dairy a day because women over fifty should.

As another aspect of nutritional fitness, we discovered simple yet healthy meals that we could eat together. We knew we wanted them to take around thirty minutes or less to prepare and stay within the guidelines of the Food Guide Pyramid while possessing the qualities of "nutritiousness and deliciousness." We have discovered meals that we prepare and eat on a regular basis. Three of them we eat every week: the flounder meal, the breakfast meal, and the hamburger and French fries meal. The others we prepare as we feel led.

Now, let's discover an eating plan for you. List below the foods that you really like and want to continue eating. To lose weight, you have three choices for these particular foods. One, eat it less often. Two, make the portions smaller. Three, find a healthier version that you still enjoy. You can actually do all three or any combination thereof.

1.   6.

2.   7.

3.   8.

4.   9.

5.   10.

List below the foods that you already know you do not like and do not want to eat.

1.   6.

2.   7.

3.   8.

4.   9.

5.   10.

Refer to the Healthy Foods list, Appendix C in your book, and circle the ones that you like or that you want to try. Strike through the ones you dislike or hate. You can experiment with the remainder. Try a new one every week.

We discovered two important concepts to keep in mind for effective weight loss. One, do not skip a meal or a snack. By eating on a regular basis, it stabilizes your metabolism, prevents hunger, and helps to control cravings. Two, remain conscious of your food choices for each meal as you plan.

Now, let's decide your snacks. Record those below.

	Morning	Afternoon	Evening
Monday			
Tuesday			
Wednesday			
Thursday			
Friday			
Saturday			
Sunday			

Next, let's decide your breakfasts. Record those below.

Monday

Tuesday

Wednesday

Thursday

Friday

Saturday

Sunday

And lastly, let's decide your lunches. Record those.

Monday

Tuesday

Wednesday

Thursday

Friday

Saturday

Sunday

Finally, let's decide your dinners. We included recipes in the book in Appendix D. Feel free to use those, surf the net, download an app, or search other places for healthy, delicious dinners that you enjoy. When you find something that you really like, please share that with others!

Monday

Tuesday

Wednesday

Thursday

Friday

Saturday

Sunday

WEEK 2: DAY 1

Memory Verse: "Now to Him who is able to do above and beyond all that we ask or think according to the power that works in us—to him be glory in the church and in Christ Jesus to all generations, forever and ever. Amen" (Eph. 3:20-21).

Challenge: This week, eat broiled or baked fish at least once.

Focus: Nutritional Fitness

NATHAN'S NOTIONS

Paul's doxology (praise to God) fills his readers with hope and cheer as they ponder the ability of God to do great things for His people. When we think of the doxology in connection with prayer, a couple of things stand out: a deep sense of need and a strong supply of hope.

Perhaps we felt reluctant to ask for God's help, especially with our deep sense of need to lose weight. We dishonor God by not asking for His help; for He remains ready, willing, and able to assist. Jesus says, "Whatever you ask in my name, I will do it so that the Father may be glorified in the Son" (John 14:13).

Ask God to help you make the right decisions about what food to eat. The Bible tells us, "Now if any of you lacks wisdom, he should ask God—who gives to all generously and ungrudgingly—and it will be given to him" (James 1:5). Our memory verse reminds us that not only can God help us in all that we ask, but even beyond all we can think! God stands ready to pour out blessings upon us, fueling a strong supply of hope. He says, "See if I will not open the floodgates of heaven and pour out a blessing for you without measure" (Mal. 3:10b).

You may already pray before you eat. Instead of reciting a nonchalant thanks for food, try this: "Dear God, I give You thanks for this food You have provided. Help me to eat only what I need to satisfy my hunger. Please help me to know when to stop, and give me the courage to put the fork down and push the plate away. I have a deep sense of my need to lose weight and a strong supply of hope that You can help me. I eat this meal in Your Name and for Your honor. In Jesus' Name, Amen."

TAMMY'S TIDBITS

When choosing fish, opt for wild over farm-raised. A wild fish has to work harder, so it has less fat and more nutritional value.

WEEK 2: DAY 2

Memory Verse: "Now to him who is able to do above and beyond all that we ask or think according to the power that works in us—to him be glory in the church and in Christ Jesus to all generations, forever and ever. Amen" (Eph. 3:20-21).

Challenge: This week, eat broiled or baked fish at least once.

Focus: Benefits of Water

NATHAN'S NOTIONS

Let's consider some implications involved with praying to God, Who exists to answer our prayers beyond what we can ask or think. If we have made prayer a daily exercise in monotony, we have disgraced the nature of God, Who loves to hear from His children and desires to meet their deepest needs. Because of this, we should feel compelled not to pray poorly or haphazardly.

Another implication calls us to remember how God answered our prayers in the past. Think of the times you needed Him, and He provided out of His grace what you required. Just as God showed His love to you in tangible ways in the past, He wants to show you His love by giving you the desire of your heart: a healthy body in which to glorify His name.

A further implication in prayer causes us to show more gratitude to God for all His tender mercies. We receive so many mercies of God, and most of them we take for granted—for instance, the simple remedy He has provided to help control pain. The benefits of water show God's mercies each and every day, including the fact that drinking the right amount of water daily helps to control muscle pain.[5]

Spend time praying in a way that honors God's desire to go beyond what you can ever ask or think. Today, remember, the only restriction of God intervening in your life to achieve success lies in your silence. Pray, asking for God's help to lose weight. Watch, as you see His power work in your life to answer your prayer. Speak, letting others know the glory of God as He helps you achieve the healthiest version of you that can exist!

TAMMY'S TIDBITS

Try increasing your water intake, and notice the different aches and pains in your muscles that begin to slowly fade away. Drink a full glass of water before each meal as a way to increase your water intake.

---

5 Steve Reynolds, *Bod4God: The Four Keys to Weight Loss* (Ventura: Regal from Gospel Light, 2009), 135.

WEEK 2: DAY 3

Memory Verse: "Now to him who is able to do above and beyond all that we ask or think according to the power that works in us—to him be glory in the church and in Christ Jesus to all generations, forever and ever. Amen" (Eph. 3:20-21).

Challenge: This week, eat broiled or baked fish at least once.

Focus: Physical Fitness

NATHAN'S NOTIONS

In today's devotion, we will consider the last words of our memory verse, *auto he doxa*, "to Him be glory."[6] We want to focus on the debt that we owe God: glory. All glory belongs to God, not just some of it.

When others begin to notice our weight dropping off, we can easily give ourselves the credit. Successful weight loss cannot happen without the grace of God; that's why we owe Him a debt of glory! When we study the amazing riches of the grace of God, it gives birth to an outburst of praise toward Him, the Divine Source of all this mercy—past, present, and future. We remember mercy in the past upon forgiveness of our sins at salvation. We cherish mercy in the present, experiencing His loving presence giving us the help we need each day. We eagerly anticipate mercy in the future, knowing our eternal destiny lies with Him! To God belongs all credit and glory for the scheme of grace and the work of grace carried out in His Son!

As we focus on physical fitness in today's devotion, we need to acknowledge the debt of glory we owe God and determine to pay that debt through every aspect of our lives. Do not take for granted the body God has given you to inhabit for a period of time here on the earth. Do not abuse your body through unhealthy eating habits or lack of physical activity. Pay your debt of glory to God by conditioning your body through exercise to operate at the most efficient manner possible.

TAMMY'S TIDBITS

Try exercising thirty minutes a day. If that seems like too much work, then just try five or ten minutes a day to start.

---

6 Kittel, 2:237-251.

WEEK 2: DAY 4

Memory Verse: "Now to him who is able to do above and beyond all that we ask or think according to the power that works in us—to him be glory in the church and in Christ Jesus to all generations, forever and ever. Amen" (Eph. 3:20-21).

Challenge: This week, eat broiled or baked fish at least once.

Challenge Checkup: Have you eaten fish yet this week? If not, make a point to do so in the next few days. You can choose from any fish you want, fixed anyway you want, except fried. Try fish just once. If you don't like it, never eat it again!

Focus: Benefits of Effective Time Management

NATHAN'S NOTIONS

Today, we will consider the period of time associated with our memory verse. To do so, we need to know how Ephesians 3:21 ends. It says, "To all generations, forever and ever. Amen." Paul uses a familiar writing technique common in the first century: a cumulative expression of great force. He writes, *eis pasas tas geneas tou aionos ton aionon. Amen.* It literally translates as "to all the generations of the age of ages. Amen."[7] This technique builds words on top of each other for special emphasis.

We, along with all of creation, will continue to give God glory during all the ages of time. Time rolls on, waiting for no one. God is as constant as time. If God did not exist forever, then time and worship of God would not last forever. The Church also exists as constant as time. The redeemed have an eternal existence in Heaven secured by the precious blood of Christ. Once we accept Jesus into our hearts, we live forever. The reasons to praise God are as constant as time, as well. His infinite excellence, His plan of redemption, His Fatherhood, and His communication of love will all last forever. When we praise God and give Him glory for His Person, power, and provisions, He enthrones Himself upon our hearts and gives us peace.

If you feel stressed over your weight loss journey, give God glory for what He has already done in your life and how He currently helps you each day. Take time today just to thank God for the body He gave you to inhabit for a few short years on this earth and tell Him you will honor and glorify His name each day as you Imagine Not as Much!

TAMMY'S TIDBITS

To not feel overwhelmed in your weight loss journey, take one day at a time. You've got this, one step at a time!

---

7 Green, 4:524.

WEEK 2: DAY 5

Memory Verse: "Now to him who is able to do above and beyond all that we ask or think according to the power that works in us—to him be glory in the church and in Christ Jesus to all generations, forever and ever. Amen" (Eph. 3:20-21).

Challenge: This week, eat broiled or baked fish at least once.

Focus: Motivational Fitness

NATHAN'S NOTIONS

Eight words capture our attention in this day's devotion: "according to the power that works in us." These words translate, *kata taen dunamin taen energoumenaen en hemin.* Note two words: *dunamin,*[8] from where we derive the English word, "dynamite," and *energoumenaen,*[9] a form of the word "energy." "Dynamite" and "energy" identify the power that we can expect from God when we pray. This power goes "above and beyond all that we ask or think!" God's power stands not only irreversibly pledged, but also irrevocably in operation in both an absolute capacity and a relative capacity.

In God's absolute capacity, He possesses the ability to do above and beyond our imaginations. Paul used an expression of great force with the phrase, *huper panta poiasai huper ek perissou,* literally translated as, "beyond all things to do beyond above."[10] Paul makes His point clear—you cannot possibly imagine more than God's power to bless you!

The nature and measure of our spiritual aspirations and cravings determines the relative capacity of God's power. His communication to penetrate our hearts and change our lives remains connected to our receptivity. God will not overrun our free will.

Choose to open yourself to the power of God. Our focus in today's devotion calls attention to motivational fitness. When your weight-loss journey gets tough, remember the power of God stands ready to help you. God loves you and wants to see you healthy. Watch as God does a marvelous work in your life helping you to achieve the goal you never thought possible!

TAMMY'S TIDBITS

By now, you may feel better and have more energy. Keep the great feeling of having more energy in your mind as motivation to successfully meet your weight loss goal!

---

8 Walter Grundmann, "The Concept of Power in the N.T.," *Theological Dictionary of the New Testament* (Grand Rapids: Wm. B. Eerdmans Publishing Company, 1964), 2:299-317.
9 Thayer, 215.
10 Green, 4:524.

WEEK 2: DAY 6

Memory Verse: "Now to him who is able to do above and beyond all that we ask or think according to the power that works in us—to him be glory in the church and in Christ Jesus to all generations, forever and ever. Amen" (Eph. 3:20-21).

Challenge: This week, eat broiled or baked fish at least once.

Focus: Benefits of Friends

NATHAN'S NOTIONS

In today's devotion, let's focus on the words at the end of our memory verse: "in the church." These words describe the sphere in which expressing God's glory should excel. Even though God calls upon everything that has breath to give Him glory, those who make up the Church have more reasons than "anything else" to do so. I use Church with a capital "C" to refer to every person who prays to invite Jesus into their heart.

God blesses us in so many ways. He saved us from our sins through the blood of His Son. He walks with us every day through the presence of His Holy Spirit. We have the amazing privilege to call Him "Our Father," as He guides us, sustains us, and lifts us up when we're down. So many reasons to give Him glory, yet so few do in the Church.

Those who find a local church in which to worship and serve Him discover deeper reasons to say, "To Him be glory." If they find a church that uplifts God in everything they do, they discover a vibrant, real, and contagious faith!

Those who find an active, local church worshiping and serving God will find a place to call home and people to call friends. These friends comprise the outward theater on which the grace of God plays to a watching world. Friends help us to accomplish more than what we could do alone. You may have tried to lose weight in the past and failed. The Imagine Not as Much support group will help you tremendously. They will help you not only to lose weight, but also to serve as a conduit to show a watching world the glory of God!

TAMMY'S TIDBITS

Find a friend who will hold you accountable. Grab that friend for your walk and tell them specifically all that God has done for you recently.

WEEK 2: DAY 7

Memory Verse: "Now to him who is able to do above and beyond all that we ask or think according to the power that works in us—to him be glory in the church and in Christ Jesus to all generations, forever and ever. Amen" (Eph. 3:20-21).

Challenge: This week, eat broiled or baked fish at least once.

Challenge Carryover: Now that you have tried eating fish at least once this week, try eating it on a regular basis; try it more often than you do now.

Focus: Spiritual Fitness

NATHAN'S NOTIONS

In today's devotion, we will look at "in Christ Jesus." The only reason we have to give God the glory due His name exists in the person of Jesus Christ.

In Him we can visibly see the glory of God. He reveals through His words and actions the moral glory of God. Jesus, in dealing with people in need of a Savior, shined the light of God's glory. Jesus exemplified God's glory in everything He did, everywhere He went, and at all times!

In Jesus Christ, we understand God's glory. Jesus inspires us to pursue God's glory, enamors us to express glory to God, and transports us to a life actively giving glory to God. Because of Jesus, we see God's glory, and we can experience God's glory. It seems only natural then that the glory due to God rests upon the person of Jesus.

Our emphasis today centers on spiritual fitness. If you have a personal relationship with Jesus Christ, you know the power behind Paul's words, "in Christ Jesus." If you have only a meager understanding of Jesus Christ, then you have not yet tapped into God's power. Begin by asking Jesus into your heart as personal Savior. Then ask Him to help you as you take the Imagine Not as Much journey. Once you experience this power of God through Jesus Christ, you will see great weight loss results, above and beyond what you can even imagine, as you dedicate your body for God's glory.

TAMMY'S TIDBITS

Just as you can reach out for help with nutritional, physical, and motivational fitness, you should not fear seeking help for spiritual fitness. Tell us your spiritual journey with *Imagine Not as Much*—whether good or bad, easy or difficult.

FIRST FOCUS: NUTRITIONAL FITNESS

"Put a knife to your throat if you have a big appetite" (Prov. 23:2).

WEEK 3: STRATEGIES

As a further aspect of nutritional fitness, consider how to handle special occasions like birthdays, holidays, and parties at work and/or with friends. Plan ahead for special occasions. Plan on enjoying yourself while eating in moderation and savoring the flavors of everything you desire. Act like Scarlet O'Hara, and eat a healthy snack or light meal before you attend. Also, plan on wearing tight-fitting clothing. If your clothes already fit snugly, you mentally will not want to make them any tighter, thus unconsciously curbing your appetite.

Also, consider planning ahead when you eat out, especially at all-you-can-eat buffets or potluck dinners. Nathan tries to remember "2 + 1 + 1 then done": two vegetables, plus one protein, plus one starch on one plate equals four servings, and then done.

Tammy chooses smaller portions of several items that would equal four servings. In that way, she does not feel deprived of some of her favorites, such as macaroni and cheese.

If you know you will possibly eat more than usual during your excursion, eat smaller, healthy meals during the day, so you can splurge a little during your event. For carry-in dinners, make sure to bring healthy options that you enjoy.

Quite honestly, eating away from home posed as Nathan's greatest challenge because he loves to eat, and he has very little self-control. However, he found something else when eating out—his happy place. When he has eaten enough to achieve happiness and contentment with his nutritional intake, he quits. He does not force himself to finish his plate. After a few times of doing this, he learned to place enough food on his plate to satisfy himself, but not too much to make him full.

Some basic nutritional tips to follow:
- Drink lots of water each day (at least 64 ounces).
- Eat grilled or broiled fish every week.
- Choose chicken more than beef on a regular basis.
- Choose frozen yogurt instead of ice cream for your sweet tooth, watching the toppings because they can add sugar and calories.
- Do not add mayonnaise to a grilled chicken sandwich for it adds unnecessary fat and calories.

- When eating salad, try a vinaigrette dressing or a fat-free or low-fat option.
- When you eat blueberries, you consume a powerful antioxidant food.
- Stay aware of your food choices.
- Eat foods high in fiber and low in calories.
- Eat foods high in protein and low in calories.
- Eat slowly, putting your fork down and taking sips of water between bites.
- When eating out at a restaurant that serves large portions, ask for a to-go box at the beginning of the meal. Divide your food in half; put it in the box; and take it home to enjoy another day.
- Take a multivitamin.
- Be sure to get enough sleep.
- Use smaller plates.

For the first few weeks, you will engage in experimentation, experimentation, and more experimentation. Don't beat yourself up if you make non-healthy food choices for a meal or a day. That does not ruin everything. Make sure to track what you eat, either by using a food journal or an app on your smartphone.

You can do it! We believe in you; and with the Lord's help, you can truly meet your weight-loss goal.

WEEK 3: DAY 1

Memory Verse: "Put a knife to your throat if you have a big appetite" (Prov. 23:2).

Challenge: This week, purposely eat between five and six times every day: three meals with two or three snacks.

Focus: Nutritional Fitness

NATHAN'S NOTIONS

Our memory verse this week falls in between two other verses making one train of thought in context. All week, we will consider Proverbs 23:1-3. The visual image of someone eating a meal with a knife to their throat makes me laugh. Solomon used the absurd—a hyperbole—to drive home the point of not making a glutton of oneself.

Nutritional fitness guides our focus today. We want to consider balancing eating the delicious food God has created with self-control. For everything that God intends for good, there always remains an opportunity for misuse and abuse, thus making it sinful. If we give in to our appetites, we let them control us instead of our controlling them.

We can enjoy all the wonderful food God has provided for us and still not have big appetites. Today and tomorrow, we will look at several things that will help strike this balance. The one for today stresses not to make any food taboo in your eating plan.

Instead of depriving yourself of your favorite food, try something different. If your favorite food constitutes something sweet, eat it only after you have eaten a healthy meal, and decide you will have only three or four bites. If a meal makes up your favorite food, then eat it on occasion and in moderation. Ask for a to-go box; cut the meal in half; and put it away for another day. Enjoy the wonderful taste with no guilt, and look forward to doing it again.

TAMMY'S TIDBITS

Start this week by planning what snacks you will have and when. Try a cup of fruit in the morning, or veggies with hummus or salsa mid-afternoon, and light Greek yogurt as a bedtime snack. Keep in mind that healthy snacks stop hunger pangs and keep you satisfied longer.

WEEK 3: DAY 2

Memory Verse: "Put a knife to your throat if you have a big appetite" (Prov. 23:2).

Challenge: This week, purposely eat between five and six times every day: three meals with two or three snacks.

Focus: Benefits of Water

NATHAN'S NOTIONS

Proverbs 23:3 guides today's devotional time. It reads, "Don't desire his choice food, for that food is deceptive." Choice, deceptive food appears as high-calorie, addictive foods that we eat without thinking. We face temptations daily. How can one strike a balance between a healthy appetite and an out-of-control appetite?

First, keep in mind what has already happened in the past with similar temptations. I remember the party my taste buds had with every bite. But I also remember my stomach pain, sluggishness, sleepiness, and guilt.

Second, keep in mind that yielding to one temptation leads to another. Some people have discovered the art of moderation. You can achieve success over choice, deceptive foods by careful planning.

Third, keep in mind that the gratification you receive from choice, deceptive foods declines with the increase of consumption. I have discovered my "happy place." I eat until I no longer experience hunger and stop when I first start feeling full. Water has helped. Drinking water before I eat increases my body's metabolism for about a half-hour, causing the body to burn twenty-five calories, helping to curb my appetite.[11]

Finally, call to mind that all excess, including food, constitutes sin. Excess misuses and profanes the body God has given us as temples of His Holy Spirit.

I pray that these suggestions will help you eat responsibly. Make a point to pay attention to all the food you eat. By not yielding to an out-of-control appetite, you defeat the deceptiveness of these foods, and you won't have to "put a knife to your throat"!

TAMMY'S TIDBITS

Sip water between every bite; it will fill you up, slow you down, and keep you from over-eating.

---

11 Zinczenko, *Eat This Not That!,* 13.

WEEK 3: DAY 3

Memory Verse: "Put a knife to your throat if you have a big appetite" (Prov. 23:2).

Challenge: This week, purposely eat between five and six times every day: three meals with two or three snacks.

Focus: Physical Fitness

NATHAN'S NOTIONS

Physical fitness guides today's devotional. The memory verse this week used an exaggeration to make a point to stop yourself from eating a lot in front of a ruler. When we carry over that point of going to the extreme, we can see the implications in taking care of our bodies. Some people try to avoid physical activity at all costs. They sit in a chair at work, then come home to sit in a chair with a remote for the TV.

A few simple yet powerful things can help to increase our level of physical activity. Make time for exercise. This may constitute a drastic step because our lives already seem crowded with "have to's." We all have the same amount of time in every day. Consider missing exercise as shortening your time of productive physical activity. Instead of considering exercise as a luxury, consider it as a necessity for promoting good health.

Find a physical activity to counteract your sedentary routines. On your breaks at work, walk around instead of sitting in a chair, or better yet, take the stairs. While watching television, alternate between walking around your house and doing a weight-lifting routine with cans from the pantry.

Think outside the box when it comes to physical activity. Make exercise a priority; make it fun; and make it creative. You never know your capabilities until you begin to stretch them! Choose to take drastic measures to incorporate daily exercise into your life. Your current body will say thank you now, and your future body will never regret it!

TAMMY'S TIDBITS

Deliberately plan physical activity with just as much dedication as you plan to eat healthy. Nathan and I have never regretted exercising, but we always regret not exercising.

WEEK 3: DAY 4

Memory Verse: "Put a knife to your throat if you have a big appetite" (Prov. 23:2).

Challenge: This week, purposely eat between five and six times every day: three meals with two or three snacks.

Challenge Check-up: Have you gotten into the habit of eating throughout the day? If you have eaten only three or fewer times a day, this challenge may present a particular difficulty for you. But keep trying until you find the right combination that works for you.

Focus: Benefits of Effective Time Management

NATHAN'S NOTIONS

Our focus on the benefits of effective time management in today's devotional will look at specific times that we need to follow the advice of our memory verse. These times typically occur on special occasions and when we go out to eat. These scenarios posed my greatest threat to losing and maintaining weight: having people over, attending special occasions, and eating out. I found a way to conquer them, and you can, too.

You can prepare to receive guests in your home by buying and preparing healthy food alternatives, along with foods people expect. Prepare to attend a special event by telling yourself how much you will consume during the celebration. You may not know the choices until you arrive, but you can eat and stay within your healthy eating plan. Plan on an enjoyable meal out focusing on the conversation and time of fellowship. Order sensibly. When the meal arrives, take your time to eat it. One of the benefits of effective time management consists of making time to eat a meal slowly—at least twenty minutes—which will help you to lose weight. Before you know it, you will have eaten a healthy meal in sensible portions and will have enjoyed time with your loved ones as well.

By following these simple guidelines, you can conquer those times that represent the most challenging obstacles to your permanent weight loss. You can practice the principles you learn every day for the rest of your life, as a lifestyle change.

TAMMY'S TIDBITS

I have three more suggestions. First, eat a snack before the event. Second, remember to wear tight-fitting clothing instead of looser apparel. Third, focus on the importance of good fellowship with family and friends, instead of the food.

WEEK 3: DAY 5

Memory Verse: "Put a knife to your throat if you have a big appetite" (Prov. 23:2).

Challenge: This week, purposely eat between five and six times every day: three meals with two or three snacks.

Focus: Motivational Fitness

NATHAN'S NOTIONS

As we focus on the phrase in our memory verse, "If you have a big appetite," in relation to motivational fitness, we want to look at some people who have inclinations for indulgence and how to stay motivated to keep those indulgences in check. I have already revealed two indulgences: eating until I felt full and a routine of a sedentary lifestyle.

I learned that I did not have to eat until I got a full feeling to satisfy my hunger. I had to convince myself that this habit of overeating had to die. I knew that if I could create a new habit based on eating healthy food in the right portions at the right times, I could stick with it.

Another habit that had to die consisted of a sedentary lifestyle. Before I started college in 1982, I had a very active life. I enjoyed working up a "good sweat." Then, I had to hit the books to earn a bachelor's degree and a master's degree. I spent seven years in my studies. Each year, my weight increased, and my level of activity decreased.

I became so accustomed to very little activity that the slightest physical effort caused breathlessness, redness in the face, and fatigue. In May of 2013, I determined that every day I would devote myself to at least one hour of physical activity. I found it hard at first, but after several days of concentrated effort, I began to form a new habit.

If you share this character trait with me—"a man given to appetite"—use it to your advantage to develop new eating routines and exercise skills. "Put a knife to your throat" on all your old, addictive, unhealthy actions. Take drastic measures to put to death all things that kept you from losing weight.

TAMMY'S TIDBITS

Keep in mind your end result. Imagine how you will feel when you meet the short-term goal that you set for yourself.

WEEK 3: DAY 6

Memory Verse: "Put a knife to your throat if you have a big appetite" (Prov. 23:2).

Challenge: This week, purposely eat between five and six times every day: three meals with two or three snacks.

Focus: Benefits of Friends

NATHAN'S NOTIONS

We will spend time today looking at another meaning of Proverbs 23:3: "Don't desire his choice food, for that food is deceptive." We will consider the reason Solomon said that choice food contains deception and what that means for us today.

King Solomon knew that when a ruler extended an act of kindness, it always came with a price. As king, he always had a purpose in mind whenever he prepared a banquet and invited guests. An invitation from him to attend a banquet had a reason, and that reason may not have had a good ending. Solomon encourages the readers of his proverbs to consider very carefully the reason they may sit at the banquet table of a ruler.

Most gatherings today have unhealthy food present. Just as food offered by a ruler comes with a price, every bite that we take without considering it carefully comes with a price. That price may reveal itself as a plateau, guilt over not making right choices, or a ravenous sweet tooth that we cannot control.

Some people act as healthy-eating saboteurs. One way to deal with them includes making sure we attend gatherings with friends who know of our commitment to healthy living. At a gathering, stick together; lean upon each other's strengths; and enjoy the event guilt-free.

Next time someone asks you to indulge, consider for a moment their motivation. Before you take that bite, remember it comes with a price. If the price is not worth it, "put a knife to your throat!"

TAMMY'S TIDBITS

Offer to help serve and/or clean up after a special occasion. That will keep you and a friend busy and away from the dreaded dessert table.

WEEK 3: DAY 7

Memory Verse: "Put a knife to your throat if you have a big appetite" (Prov. 23:2).

Challenge: This week, purposely eat between five and six times every day: three meals with two or three snacks.

Challenge Carryover: Make a practice of eating often throughout each day for the rest of your life. You will experience the surprising benefits of eating less while avoiding hunger.

Focus: Spiritual Fitness

NATHAN'S NOTIONS

Today's focus on spiritual fitness considers Proverbs 23:1: "When you sit down to dine with a ruler, consider carefully what is before you." Our thoughts will center on the wisdom in depending upon God instead of people in power.

When you depend upon people in power, you place yourself in a dangerous predicament. You put yourself under their power and influence. They not only have the power to help you, they also possess the power to harm you. You face temptation to stoop to unworthy actions. You consider doing things that had never entered your mind. You lose self-reliance. You become obsessed with pleasing this person. You live in constant fear of falling out of favor. You consider carefully what you say and do.

Let's look at the difference in depending upon God instead of on an earthly ruler. When you depend upon God, you put yourself under His power and influence. He has the power to help you through each day, and He has the ability to influence you to make the right decisions. You stay focused on living your life in a way that honors and glorifies God. You make decisions based upon the truth of God's Word, the leadership of the Holy Spirit, and the inspiration of Jesus living in your heart. You gain self-reliance as you depend upon God to meet your needs. Pleasing Him becomes your focus. You live your life with no fear. You will never experience falling out of favor with God.

Your weight-loss journey serves as a way to please God. The more you make a habit of curbing your appetite, the less often you will visualize "putting a knife to your throat" to make wise, healthy decisions.

TAMMY'S TIDBITS

It takes enormous strength to say no to decadent foods. It takes enormous courage to tell a friend, "No, thank you." Stand firm in the faith that you've got this; you can lose weight!

SECOND FOCUS: PHYSICAL FITNESS

"Therefore, brothers and sisters, in view of the mercies of God, I urge you to present your bodies as a living sacrifice, holy and pleasing to God; this is your true worship" (Rom. 12:1).

WEEK 4: PHYSICAL ACTIVITY

In the beginning of your exercise journey, try to do at least three to four days a week for as long as you can, building up to twenty to thirty minutes a day. One must include physical fitness to lose weight and maintain a healthy body. Eventually, spend at least one hour a day, six days a week, doing some type of physical fitness. We recommend to begin with aerobic activity for the first few weeks until some of the weight begins to fall off. After a while, when you have conditioned your heart and lungs, add anaerobic activity. The American College of Sports Medicine (ACSM) developed the acronym FITT as a good formula to determine your level of physical activity.[12]

F = Frequency   The number of days per week you will exercise.

I = Intensity   The level of stress you will put your body through as you exercise.

T = Time   How much time you will exercise each day.

T = Type   Aerobic, anaerobic, or lifestyle.

The higher your FITT number, the greater your fitness level. Your **F**requency number can range between zero days to seven days. We recommend no more than six days to give your body a day of rest.

Your **I**ntensity number can fluctuate between "couch potato" and "Olympic athlete training." We suggest an intensity level that challenges you physically without putting yourself in danger of injury, heart attack, or stroke.

Your **T**ime number can vary between zero minutes each day to an all-day marathon of activity. We propose starting at what you can do and extending your exercise time on regular intervals until you reach one hour a day. Your body can achieve physical fitness with an hour of exercise each day. If you go beyond an hour a day, make sure that you have a good reason, like training for a special event. Also, consult a doctor before beginning any exercise program.

Your **T**ype number can span between zero and three: aerobic, anaerobic, and lifestyle. We will cover the first two types in the following two chapters. Incorporating lifestyle physical activity simply means transforming your daily activities into something more physically challenging. Examples include doing leg lifts while cooking dinner, walking in place during

---

12 Barbara Bushman, Editor, *American College of Sports Medicine Complete Guide to Fitness & Health: Physical Activity and Nutrition Guidelines for Every Age (Champaign: Human Kinetics, 2011)*, 320-323.

commercials, parking farther away from the front door of your favorite store, or taking the stairs a flight or two instead of the elevator. By using your imagination, you can create many more lifestyle physical activities!

Now, how do we fit in physical fitness? We start with aerobic and anaerobic exercise first thing in the morning. We get up at 5:00 am Monday through Friday and do one hour of exercise. We call Saturday a "no alarm day" and just rise when we naturally wake to do our one-hour exercise. We often change things up a bit with the type and kinds of exercise we do. We go to bed early, so we can continue to get a good night's sleep. It has become so important to us, very little keeps us from exercising together in the mornings.

How do we fit in lifestyle physical activity? Nathan, in his job as pastor, takes the stairs instead of the elevators at the hospitals when he visits patients. Tammy purposely parks on the third floor of the parking garage, walking up two flights of steps at the end of her work day.

Where can you fit in an hour of exercise? Remember, smaller sections of time work just as well if an hour block of time does not work for you. Try a half-hour in the morning and a half-hour in the evening.

Record your time for exercise on a regular basis in the space below:

Monday

Tuesday

Wednesday

Thursday

Friday

Saturday

Sunday   Rest

Record the different types of physical activities you will incorporate into your lifestyle:

WEEK 4: DAY 1

Memory Verse: "Therefore, brothers and sisters, in view of the mercies of God, I urge you to present your bodies as a living sacrifice, holy and pleasing to God; this is your true worship" (Rom. 12:1).

Challenge: This week, exercise for a least thirty minutes every day, and track your activity.

Focus: Physical Fitness

NATHAN'S NOTIONS

In their devotion to God, Christians will consecrate their bodies as agents of spiritual ministry. If we renew and purify our spirits through a relationship with Jesus, our actions will clearly show it. We choose how to use our bodies—either as implements of sin or instruments for righteousness. Paul puts it this way, "Therefore do not let sin reign in your mortal body, so that you obey its desires. And do not offer any parts of it to sin as weapons for unrighteousness. But as those who are alive from the dead, offer yourselves to God, and all the parts of yourselves to God as weapons for righteousness" (Rom. 6:12-13).

The word used in Romans 6:13 repeats in our memory verse this week, *parastesai*, meaning "offer, present."[13] The Greek translation of the Hebrew Old Testament, called the Septuagint, uses this word to refer to the presentation of sacrificial animals at God's altar. We each sacrifice our eyes to God to read His Word and survey His work in creation instead of fulfilling our lusts. We each sacrifice our ears to God to hear swiftly His instruction and His voice and purposely to tune out gossip. We each sacrifice our hands to God to help someone in need. We each sacrifice our feet to God to go where He wants us to go. We each sacrifice our mouths to God so that we speak with grace seasoned with salt and not with corrupt communication. We each sacrifice our bodies to do God's work in accordance with His will.

In Rome, during Paul's lifetime, people abused their bodies in fulfilling their lustful desires. He wrote, "Therefore God delivered them over in the desires of their hearts to sexual impurity, so that their bodies were degraded among themselves" (Rom. 1:24). The practice of sexual impurity prevails today. Instead of abusing your body, choose to sacrifice your body to God. Determine to develop it in the best way possible through daily exercise for God to use as long as you live upon this earth.

TAMMY'S TIDBITS

Think about what time of day you want to exercise. Plan how much time you will spend on exercise. Start with what you can do, and slowly build up.

---

13 Bo Reicke and George Bertram, "*paristami,paristano* in Non-Biblical Greek, Septuagint, and The New Testament" in *Theological Dictionary of the New Testament* (Grand Rapids: Wm. B. Eerdmans Publishing Company, 1967), 5:837-841.

WEEK 4: DAY 2

Memory Verse: "Therefore, brothers and sisters, in view of the mercies of God, I urge you to present your bodies as a living sacrifice, holy and pleasing to God; this is your true worship" (Rom. 12:1).

Challenge: This week, exercise for a least thirty minutes every day, and track your activity.

Focus: Benefits of Water

NATHAN'S NOTIONS

The heart, or seat of emotions, stands alone as the most important part of our body to present to God as a sacrifice. Whatever seems important in our hearts, we will accomplish. God gave us emotions to help us express ourselves in different situations. When we present our emotions to God as sacrifices, we say to Him, "You have the right to rule our hearts." The emotions that we connect with our desires will carry us on to succeed.

Let's take drinking water as an example. God has designed our bodies to receive pure and simple water as the best liquid for hydration. In addition, not drinking enough water increases fat deposits, stopping their metabolizing into energy. So, drinking water decreases fat deposits![14]

If we want to lose weight and do not like drinking water, then we need to specifically pray that God will place in our hearts a desire to drink water. I still have an old nature as a part of me that will never leave until I see Jesus in Heaven. That old nature will choose a sugared soda to satisfy my thirst because of its sweetness and chemical high. However, with a relationship with Jesus, a new nature exists. The nature I feed the most becomes the one expressed out of the emotion of my heart. I feed my selfish nature when I only satisfy my immediate lust, regardless of the consequences. I feed my new nature in Christ when I satisfy Him in all I say and do. I choose water. Which desire will you choose today?

TAMMY'S TIDBITS

Keep hydrated with water when exercising.

---

14 Reynolds, *Bod4God*, 85.

WEEK 4: DAY 3

Memory Verse: "Therefore, brothers and sisters, in view of the mercies of God, I urge you to present your bodies as a living sacrifice, holy and pleasing to God; this is your true worship" (Rom. 12:1).

Challenge: This week, exercise for a least thirty minutes every day, and track your activity.

Focus: Motivational Fitness

NATHAN'S NOTIONS

Paul used a gentle and affectionate persuasion for the Christians at Rome: "Brothers . . . I urge you." He could have used forceful language demanding that they present their bodies as a sacrifice. Instead, he chose a term of affection—"brothers and sisters"—and a term of persuasion—"urge"—treating them as fellow servants. Through this gentle persuasion, Paul trusted that they would respond of their own free will to the mercies of God in Jesus Christ. The word Paul uses, *oiktirmon,* translates as, "compassion."[15] Some scholars have translated this word as "mercies," an outward expression of the compassion of God. God's mercies motivate us to give back to Him. We cannot meditate on the many, varied, suited-to-our-personal-needs, unfailing mercies of God without acknowledging their great claim upon us.

Nowhere else does the mercy of God demonstrate more clearly than in the cross of Calvary. God has provided salvation as a free gift by one's simply accepting what He did on the cross as payment for their sin debt. God "made the One who did not know sin to be sin for us, so that in him we might become the righteousness of God" (2 Cor. 5:21). One can describe God's mercies as undeserved, Sovereign, and free. God has chosen to grant eternal life and abundant life to those who will just follow Him. He has given everything for me. Out of gratitude, how can I not give back to Him a sacrifice of my body? This simple truth motivates me to sacrifice each and every day. How about you?

TAMMY'S TIDBITS

Exercise produces endorphins, a chemical reaction in your brain which creates euphoria. Endorphins clear your mind, make you feel good, and motivate you to want to exercise again.

---

15 Rudolf Bultmann, "*oiktiro, oiktirmos, oiktirmon* in Greek Usage, *oiktiro* etc. in the LXX and Judaism, *oiktipo* etc.in Primitive Christian Writings," *Theological Dictionary of the New Testament* (Grand Rapids: Wm. B. Eerdmans Publishing Company, 1967), 5:159-161.

WEEK 4: DAY 4

Memory Verse: "Therefore, brothers and sisters, in view of the mercies of God, I urge you to present your bodies as a living sacrifice, holy and pleasing to God; this is your true worship" (Rom. 12:1).

Challenge: This week, exercise for a least thirty minutes every day and track your activity.

Challenge Check-up: How many days have you exercised this week and for how long? Have you pinpointed the reasons why you did not exercise on the days you missed? Try very hard on these last few days to make a concentrated effort to give God at least thirty minutes in daily activity conditioning your body for His use.

Focus: Benefits of Effective Time Management

NATHAN'S NOTIONS

Paul urged his brothers in Christ to present their bodies as a "living sacrifice." One word he uses—*zosan* ("living")—translates to the word for life that describes a full and abundant life available only through a relationship with Jesus.[16] We can live our lives to the fullest because of the peace and joy in our hearts.

The other word Paul uses—*thusian*—translates as "sacrifice."[17] In the oldest records of nations upon the earth, sacrifice emerges as part of religious expression. Sacrifices on the part of the Jews and the heathen during Old Testament times existed for one of two reasons: either as an offering or as a propitiation, which means a substitution. We know that Jesus embodies the only propitiation sacrifice as the only substitution for our sins. Since we cannot serve as a substitute—only Jesus can—the word Paul uses to encourage us to sacrifice our bodies means "an offering to God."[18]

The Septuagint uses the word *thusian* for the burnt sacrifice, meaning we owe God for His mercies, and thus we offer Him everything.[19] People brought live animals to the altar for the burnt sacrifice to slay before the offering. As a living sacrifice, you must willingly and openly die to self on God's altar. That includes the use of time. When you die to self, you give God

---

16 Rudolf Bultmann, "The Concept of Life in the N.T.," *Theological Dictionary of the New Testament* (Grand Rapids: Wm. B. Eerdmans Publishing Company, 1964), 2:861-875.
17 Johannes Behm, "*thuo, thusia, thusiastariov* Linguistic and The Concept of Sacrifice in the New Testament" *Theological Dictionary of the New Testament* (Grand Rapids: Wm. B. Eerdmans Publishing Company, 1965), 3:180-183.
18 Behm, "*thuo, thusia, thusiastariov* Linguistic and The Concept of Sacrifice in the New Testament" *Theological Dictionary of the New Testament*, 3:180-183.
19 Behm, "*thuo, thusia, thusiastariov* Linguistic and The Concept of Sacrifice in the New Testament" *Theological Dictionary of the New Testament*, 3:184-190.

the right and freedom to use your time however He chooses. Determine that you will sacrifice your time to God. Unless you die to self first, you cannot offer your body as a living sacrifice. When you hold anything back from God, it shows an unwillingness to sacrifice.

TAMMY'S TIDBITS

Contemplate your daily schedule to determine what activities you will sacrifice to make time for exercise.

WEEK 4: DAY 5

Memory Verse: "Therefore, brothers and sisters, in view of the mercies of God, I urge you to present your bodies as a living sacrifice, holy and pleasing to God; this is your true worship."

Challenge: This week, exercise for a least thirty minutes every day and track your activity.

Focus: Spiritual Fitness

NATHAN'S NOTIONS

We have two words to study in today's devotional: *logiken*,[20] "spiritual" or "reasonable," and *latreian*,[21] "worship" or "service." *Logiken* occurs only twice in the New Testament: in our memory verse this week and in 1 Peter 2:2: "Like newborn infants, desire the pure milk of the word, so that you may grow up into your salvation." This word represents a rational, moral, spiritual serving of God, much like Jesus described to the Samaritan woman: "God is spirit, and those who worship Him must worship in Spirit and in truth" (John 4:24). It stands in direct contrast to mechanical acts of outward worship indicative of a dead heart.

Latreian appears in the Septuagint to refer to ceremonial worship of the Old Testament, especially in reference to the Passover. The counterpart to this ceremonial worship in the New Testament represents a life devoted to serving God. Paul adopts this when he says, "God is my witness, whom I serve with my spirit in telling the good news about his Son" (Rom. 1:9a).

What happens when we look at these two words together? We see the truth that spiritual worship or reasonable service presents our bodies outwardly as an act of worship in our hearts. Obedience rises to the highest and most sacred act of worship as an expression of a heart full of love for God, free from mechanical and formalistic going through the motions. We no longer embody dull lumps of clay, but serve as illuminated temples with the flame of Christ's love. Further, we express this worship personally, not through a representative. We express to God praise and give Him worship ourselves for what He has done specifically in our lives. Those who choose to offer their bodies as a living sacrifice perform this act of spiritual worship. Those who do not offer their bodies display themselves as either unreasonable, indefensible, disobedient, self-destructive, or any combination thereof. If we choose, we can use exercise as a spiritual, worshipful experience.

---

20 H.W. Heidland, "*logizomai, logismos* The Word Group in the New Testament" *Theological Dictionary of the New Testament* (Grand Rapids: Wm. B. Eerdmans Publishing Company, 1967), 4:286-292.
21 H. Strathmann, "*latreuo* and *latreia* in the New Testament," *Theological Dictionary of the New Testament* (Grand Rapids: Wm. B. Eerdmans Publishing Company, 1967), 4:62-65.

TAMMY'S TIDBITS

Think of your exercise as a living sacrifice to give honor and glory to God—especially when you don't feel like it, because that makes it a true sacrifice.

WEEK 4: DAY 6

Memory Verse: "Therefore, brothers and sisters, in view of the mercies of God, I urge you to present your bodies as a living sacrifice, holy and pleasing to God; this is your true worship" (Rom. 12:1).

Challenge: This week, exercise for a least thirty minutes every day and track your activity.

Focus: Benefits of Friends

NATHAN'S NOTIONS

We need to love God more than anything else upon this earth. Do not love other things less; just love God more. He sacrificed the most important thing to Him, His Son Jesus Christ. We will never adequately know the height of love or depth of sacrifice that it took for God the Father to send His Son to Earth, knowing He would die a cruel death on the cross. Seeing His willingness and ability to sacrifice so much for us, we can at least sacrifice our affections for Him. He deserves our best.

Our friends can help us in these acts of sacrifice. When we tell them we have started the Imagine Not as Much weight-loss journey as a way to honor God with our bodies, they can help us not to get lost in the details but to make the best use of details. Our friends can remind us, "Hey, you do all this to honor God because He deserves your highest affection!"

Once we decide to sacrifice our affections to God, we may think we have little that we can offer Him because He has given so greatly and so freely to us. We need to remember the little boy with five loaves and two fishes that he offered to Jesus. When Jesus took from the boy what he had, He blessed and multiplied it, feeding over five thousand people! When we offer God everything we have, even in a meager and feeble state, God sees it as precious in His sight.

TAMMY'S TIDBITS

I find it easier to exercise when I have someone who will exercise with me. If no one in your immediate circle will exercise with you, perhaps someone in the Imagine Not as Much group has the same issue, and you can exercise together.

WEEK 4: DAY 7

Memory Verse: "Therefore, brothers and sisters, in view of the mercies of God, I urge you to present your bodies as a living sacrifice, holy and pleasing to God; this is your true worship" (Rom. 12:1).

Challenge: This week, exercise for a least thirty minutes every day and track your activity.

Challenge Carryover: Now that you have tried to exercise at least thirty minutes each day this week, make a daily ritual of physical activity. Do something that will get you out of your chair and moving.

Focus: Nutritional Fitness

NATHAN'S NOTIONS

Today, I want to focus on the truth that offering our bodies as a living sacrifice constitutes holiness and pleases God. As stated on day four, the word that Paul uses for sacrifice connects with the burnt offering of the Old Testament. The animals presented for sacrifice had to appear without blemish. This simple fact impressed upon the worshipers the holiness of the God to whom they sacrificed. In addition, the priests who offered the sacrifices had to possess holiness as ceremonially clean.

Let's consider nutritional fitness as a practical way of presenting the very best of our bodies in a holy manner that pleases God. God embodies holiness and deserves a holy sacrifice. Everything that we eat has consequences. Some foods we consume offer very little in return for their calories, like sugared sodas. They have very little nutritive value and serve as a perfect example of empty calories.

Too much food also creates bad consequences. The amount of food we eat can cause sluggishness and unfocused thinking, making it very difficult to serve God effectively.

However, we can eat in a holy manner that pleases God. When we eat the right amount of the right kind of food at the right times, we will have the energy to serve God throughout the entire day without being sluggish, unfocused, and stuffed. I urge you this week and beyond, determine that what you place in your mouth achieves an act of spiritual worship, a holy sacrifice, pleasing to God!

TAMMY'S TIDBITS

Try eating a high protein snack just before you exercise to optimize nutritional fitness during physical activity.

SECOND FOCUS: PHYSICAL FITNESS

"I am able to do all things through him who strengthens me" (Phil. 4:13).

WEEK 5: AEROBIC EXERCISE

Aerobic activity includes any movement that increases your resting heart rate from at least fifty-five percent to eighty-five percent of the maximum heart rate. Only activity that sustains a heart rate between fifty-five to eighty-five percent of the maximum heart rate for at least ten minutes qualifies as aerobic. A normal resting heart rate for someone sitting or lying down and calm registers between sixty and one hundred beats per minute. Make sure to consult with your doctor before starting any exercise program.

Let's determine your current resting heart rate.

Take your pulse and record it: _____

Let's determine your maximum heart rate.

For men, 220 beats per minute minus your age reveals your maximum heart rate. For women, 226 beats per minute minus your age reveals your maximum heart rate.

Record your maximum heart rate: _____

Now, multiply your maximum heart rate by fifty-five percent and then again by eighty-five percent. This will give you the range of your target heart rate to reach when doing aerobic exercises.

55%:_____

85%:_____

We must stress the importance of maintaining your target heart rate for at least twenty minutes in your exercise routine. For a typical one-hour aerobic workout, we recommend ten minutes of warm-up, forty minutes of activity within the target heart rate, and ten minutes of cool-down. We must also stress the necessity of including both warm-up time and cool-down time to avoid injury.

Refer to the choices on the following page for aerobic activities. Circle the ones that you like or want to try. Strike through the ones you dislike or hate. Experiment with the remaining activities.

AEROBIC ACTIVITIES

Calories per hour for a 150-pound person

At the Gym

Elliptical Trainer	Light	544
	Moderate	680
	Vigorous	816
Stair Stepper		612
Stationary Bike	Light	374
	Moderate	476
	Vigorous	714
Rowing Machine	Light	238
	Moderate	476
	Vigorous	578
Circuit Training		544
Walking	@ 3.0	224
	@ 3.5	258
	@ 4.0	340
Running	@ 5.0	544
	@ 6.0	680
	@ 7.0	782
Interval Training		544
Plyometrics High Impact		476

Household Chores

Vacuuming	238
Scrubbing floors	258
Washing windows	204
Mopping	238
Painting	204
Moving furniture	408
Raking	292
Gardening	272
Cleaning the gutters	340

Washing the car		204
Mowing the lawn, push		374
Shoveling snow		408
Sweeping		272
Cleaning garage		404
Heavy landscaping		306

The Great Outdoors

Cycling	Leisure	272
Hiking Cross-Country		408
Snowshoeing		544
Downhill skiing	Light	340
	Moderate	408
Skiing Water		408
Rock climbing		544
Jogging		476
Rollerblading		816
Paddling canoe	Pleasure	238
Nordic walking		400
Surfing		204
Swimming	Leisure	408
Water jogging		544
Skateboarding		340
Ice skating		476

Sports

Tennis	476
Flag football	544
Driving range	204
Soccer	476
Ice Hockey	544
Basketball	544
Lacrosse	544
Boxing, punching bag	408

Tai Chi		272
Kickboxing		680
Kickball		476
Karate		680
Jiu-jitsu		680
Racquetball	Casual	476

Group Classes

Spinning	Light	476
	Moderate	714
	Vigorous	850
Step Aerobics		578
Jazzercise		408
Zumba		408
Salsa dancing		408
Dance classes		408
Cardio kickboxing		680
Water aerobics		272
Hang Gliding		238
Hip hop dance	Light	408
	Vigorous	544
Skiing Cross-Country		544

Play Time

Walking the dog		204
Playing with kids	Light	190
Dodgeball		340
Tag		224
Hula hooping		340
Jump rope		680
Skipping		680
Hopscotch		340
Jumping jacks		544
Trampoline jumping		306

If you choose walking, we have included three routines for walking inside your house during inclement weather, timed for sixty minutes, forty-five minutes, and thirty minutes. See below a description of the sixty-minute walking routine movements.

- The **numbers** correspond to time on a stopwatch. Each exercise lasts for one minute, until you start walking for ten minutes at a time.
- The first eleven exercises serve as a **warm-up**, so do them gently.
- **Walk** simply means walking in place.
- To **start**, warm up by walking in place at a slow rhythm, just bringing your feet off the floor a little, with limited swinging of your arms.
- **Kick-outs:** Place your hands on your hips, and then kick your right foot out with your heel touching the floor. Bring that foot in, and then repeat with the left foot.
- **Side-to-side:** Place your hands on your hips, then step horizontally to the right, followed by your left foot touching your right foot. Repeat in the opposite direction, stepping to the left horizontally with your right foot touching the left one.
- **Lunge forward:** Place your hands on your hips. Step forward with your right foot and bend your knee; then bring both feet back together. Repeat with the left foot.
- **Lunge backward:** Place your hands on your hips. Step backward with your right foot, bending your left knee, then bringing both feet back together. Repeat with the left foot.
- **Squats:** Place your hands on your hips. Lower your body as far as you comfortably can until your legs are perpendicular to your waist. Stand up straight and repeat.
- **All four:** Lunge forward with one leg at a time; then move your right leg out horizontally; then move your left leg out horizontally. Lunge backward with one leg at a time; then do a squat. Repeat as often as you can until the time changes.
- **Jump rope:** Extend arms out; move them in a circular motion, while lifting your feet slightly—first right, then left. You will look like someone jumping rope with an invisible rope.
- **Walk on minute twelve:** At this point onward in the walking, increase your intensity, pushing your comfort level while increasing your heart rate.
- **Side-to-side / Arms:** Repeat the side-to-side movement, but this time, do it more intensely while swinging your arms back and forth.
- **Walk for ten minutes:** We typically do not walk in place during this time, but rather walk throughout the house to break up the monotony. During this period

of extended walking, try to lift your knees as high as you can while pumping your arms as hard as you can without injuring yourself.

- **Shuffle:** Lift your feet behind you off the floor just a little, increasing the cardio impact to almost a jog.

- **Jog:** While in place, lift your legs behind you as a far as you can, almost to a run. This will further increase the intensity of your cardio.

- When doing the **repeated movements** described earlier starting at **minute twenty-nine**, increase your intensity to as much as you can stand.

- **Slow walk:** Begin your cool-down by slowing the pace of your walking in place, until you eventually lift your knees just a little and swing your arms only slightly.

- **Quad stretch:** Stand still. Lift your right leg behind you and hold with your hand for thirty seconds. Repeat with the left leg.

- **Calf stretch:** Stand still. Extend your right leg out for thirty seconds, pushing your heel down into the floor while stretching your toes upward. Repeat with the left leg.

- **Cat stretch:** Bend over to touch your toes with your fingers—or as far as you can. Slowly move your upper body until you reach the standing position. Then lift your hands over your head and stretch like a cat after a good nap.

WALKING FOR SIXTY MINUTES

0. Walk
1. Kick outs
2. Walk
3. Side to side
4. Walk
5. Lunge forward
6. Walk
7. Lunge backward
8. Walk
9. Squats
10. Walk
11. All four
12. Walk
13. Jump rope
14. Walk
15. Side to side with arms
16. Walk
17. Walk
18. Walk
19. Walk
20. Walk
21. Walk
22. Walk
23. Walk
24. Walk
25. Walk
26. Shuffle
27. Jog
28. Walk
29. Kick outs
30. Walk
31. Side to side
32. Walk
33. Lunge forward
34. Walk
35. Lunge backward
36. Walk
37. Squats
38. Walk
39. All four
40. Walk
41. Jump rope
42. Side to side with arms
43. Walk
44. Walk
45. Walk
46. Walk
47. Walk
48. Walk
49. Walk
50. Walk
51. Walk
52. Walk
53. Shuffle
54. Jog
55. Walk
56. Slow walk
57. Quad stretch
58. Calf stretch
59. Cat stretch
60. Done

WALKING FOR FORTY-FIVE MINUTES

0.	Walk	25.	Side-to-side with arms
1.	Kick-outs	26.	Walk
2.	Walk	27.	Jump rope
3.	Side-to-side	28.	Walk
4.	Walk	29.	Walk
5.	Lunge forward	30.	Walk
6.	Walk	31.	Walk
7.	Lunge backward	32.	Walk
8.	Walk	33.	Walk
9.	Squats	34.	Walk
10.	Walk	35.	Walk
11.	Walk	36.	Walk
12.	Walk	37.	Walk
13.	Walk	38.	Shuffle
14.	Walk	39.	Jog
15.	Walk	40.	Walk
16.	Walk	41.	Slow walk
17.	Walk	42.	Quad stretch
18.	Walk	43.	Calf stretch
19.	Walk	44.	Cat stretch
20.	Shuffle	45.	Done
21.	Jog		
22.	Walk		
23.	Kick-outs		
24.	Walk		

WALKING FOR THIRTY MINUTES

0.	Walk		16.	Walk
1.	Kick-outs		17.	Walk
2.	Walk		18.	Walk
3.	Side-to-side		19.	Walk
4.	Walk		20.	Walk
5.	Lunge forward		21.	Walk
6.	Walk		22.	Walk
7.	Lunge backward		23.	Shuffle
8.	Walk		24.	Jog
9.	Squats		25.	Walk
10.	Walk		26.	Slow walk
11.	Side-to-side with arms		27.	Quad stretch
12.	All three		28.	Calf stretch
13.	Walk		29.	Cat stretch
14.	Walk		30.	Done
15.	Walk			

WEEK 5: DAY 1

Memory Verse: "I am able to do all things through him who strengthens me" (Phil. 4:13).

Challenge: Each day this week, take the stairs instead of the elevator for as many floors as possible without over-exertion.

Focus: Physical Fitness

NATHAN'S NOTIONS

Today, let's consider "I am able to do all things" from our memory verse. We in no way claim the ability to do all things as God does; we simply have the strength to do all things that accompany us as humans—all things God expects of us.

The word Paul uses, *endunamounti,* translates as "empowering, strengthens."[22] Our English word "dynamite" comes from the root of this Greek word. We have the ability to do all things within the realm of our strength. Paul encourages us with the fact that we have access to much more strength than we ever thought possible.

Our strength arises out of the presence of the Lord Jesus to sustain us. Paul says it this way: "But he said to me, 'My grace is sufficient for you, for my power is perfected in weakness.' Therefore, I will most gladly boast all the more about my weaknesses, so that Christ's power may reside in me" (2 Cor. 12:9). When we turn our weaknesses over to the Lord, they become strengths, and we discover we can do all things through Him.

In relation to physical fitness, we want you to challenge yourself. The official challenge encourages you to take the stairs instead of the elevator. Try something new in physical activity, or push yourself to a new limit in an old physical activity. Before you say "I can't" or "that's impossible," remember our memory verse.

In your *Imagine Not as Much* journey, do not base your level of physical activity or your weight-loss goal simply on what you think you can achieve. Imagine greater. Do as much as you can for as long as you can knowing that God wants to help you succeed. Then you can say, "I am able to do all things through Him who strengthens me."

TAMMY'S TIDBITS

Take one flight of steps today. If you have already accomplished that, then add an additional flight this week.

---

22 Grundmann, 2:299-317.

WEEK 5: DAY 2

Memory Verse: "I am able to do all things through him who strengthens me."

Challenge: Each day this week, take the stairs instead of the elevator for as many floors as possible without over-exertion.

Focus: Benefits of Water

NATHAN'S NOTIONS

In today's devotion, we want to look at the source of our strength, Jesus Christ. Our memory verse simply has "him." The pronoun "him" refers back to Philippians 4:10a, which states, "I rejoiced in the Lord." If we have to rely on our own power for the ability to do things, our efforts would fall miserably short. But our power does not rest upon ourselves; it rests upon Jesus Christ.

Jesus provides our Source of strength with an inspiration of Divine energy. Paul points to a tangible, live Person Who inspires strength—not a mere sense of courage swelling from one's inside. Jesus carries with Him a positive outflow of God's Spirit to everyone who has a personal relationship with Him.

Our focus today highlights the benefits of drinking water. You have the opportunity and joy through Jesus to encounter Him as the Living Water of Life (John 7:37-39). You also have the ability of drinking sufficient amounts of physical water to achieve successful, permanent weight loss!

Jesus Christ strengthens us by the very fact of His union with us. We cannot simply know about Jesus for His power to flow into us and through us; we have to know Jesus intimately by inviting Him into our hearts as our personal Lord and Savior. Jesus Christ strengthens us as we exercise our faith in Him. We receive the power that Christ has to offer in direct proportion to the level of our faith. The energy that provides our strength does not rest in our faith per se, but rather in the One in Whom our faith abides, Jesus Christ. Still, faith remains as the channel through which God has designed Christ's power to flow.

We consistently see God meeting our needs by providing strength that we did not know existed. He intervenes in our lives to help us succeed each day. Because of these two facts, we can come to a place of peace in our hearts, knowing that He will do it again tomorrow.

TAMMY'S TIDBITS

Try drinking eight ounces of water before and after you exercise. This will help energize you and replenish you.

WEEK 5: DAY 3

Memory Verse: "I am able to do all things through him who strengthens me."

Challenge: Each day this week, take the stairs instead of the elevator for as many floors as possible without over-exertion.

Focus: Motivational Fitness

NATHAN'S NOTIONS

We will focus on motivational fitness in today's devotional. One thing that should motivate us comes through in a summary of our memory verse: Christians exhibit strong souls.

We, like Paul, can embrace the role of genuine reformers as strong souls. Paul's reformation targeted the inner man. Through his life, he spent his time introducing people to the Lord Jesus. Paul knew the truth that as he did the Father's work of reformation, He would grant him the strength through Jesus to accomplish more than he could ever imagine. Just think for a moment about the influence this one person, Paul, had on the world.

Today, embrace the truth that you possess a strong soul as a born-again believer. Make a conscious effort to reform the world around you—not through your own talent or strength, but in Jesus, Who strengthens you.

You can achieve motivational fitness as you embrace the truth of our memory verse. Because of your personal relationship with Jesus, you have the ability to do the work of a reformer. View your weight loss journey as a way to impact and reform the people in your life. As they notice your healthy eating habits and increased physical activity, point them to Jesus, Who gives you the strength to continue until you reach your goal. Invite them to join you on the journey.

TAMMY'S TIDBITS

Forgive yourself for your weaknesses. Remind yourself that God has given you strength and, in turn, motivation. He won't quit now. On days that you struggle in this journey, look back at another time of struggle, and remember, you can overcome!

WEEK 5: DAY 4

Memory Verse: "I am able to do all things through him who strengthens me" (Phil. 4:13).

Challenge: Each day this week, take the stairs instead of the elevator for as many floors as possible without over-exertion.

Challenge Check-up: How many flights of stairs have you taken this week as compared to what you normally climb? For the remainder of the week, try to take just one more flight of stairs than you have already completed.

Focus: Benefits of Effective Time Management

NATHAN'S NOTIONS

In today's devotion, we will consider one of the reasons why Jesus grants us the strength to do all things. He gives us strength to fulfill the duties that He calls us to do.

We find our duties from the Bible. When critics attack its veracity, we can stay strong as we point them to the many prophetic passages in the Old Testament about the Messiah that Jesus fulfilled. The Old Testament contains 456 specific prophecies of the Messiah, and Jesus fulfills each one of them. In a study done by David Williams and Peter Stone, the chance of one person fulfilling eight prophecies is one in 10^{17} power (seventeen zeroes). They also calculated the odds that one man could fulfill forty-eight of the specific prophecies and came up with one in 10157 power. Jesus actually fulfilled 456 of them.[23]

In fulfilling our duty, we can seek God's help and strength. In our focus on effective time management, take time to acquire the skills for weight loss. You will continue to receive information through the thirteen-week class and the book. Take time to gain the skills necessary to achieve permanent weight loss. Learn how to read labels; how to count calories; and how to buy, cook, and eat healthy foods. Learn how your body moves and the best aerobic and anaerobic exercises that work for you. You can acquire the skills necessary to fulfill your dream of a healthy body. Because of your faith in Jesus, you can bear the heaviest burden and accomplish the hardest task.

TAMMY'S TIDBITS

Make it your duty to plan for the day: what you will eat, when you will exercise, and what time you will do the next devotion.

---

23 GBFan, "The Mathematical Probability of Jesus Christ," HouseofPolitics.com, houseofpolitics.com/threads/the-mathematical-probability-of-jesus-christ.17647 (accessed July 18, 2015).

WEEK 5: DAY 5

Memory Verse: "I am able to do all things through him who strengthens me" (Phil. 4:13).

Challenge: Each day this week, take the stairs instead of the elevator for as many floors as possible without over exertion.

Focus: Spiritual Fitness

NATHAN'S NOTIONS

As we consider spiritual fitness, we will look at how Jesus came to have strength to give. We want to discover how Jesus qualified as the "him who strengthens me."

The work set before Jesus required strength. Jesus constantly did the work God gave Him to do as Savior. In fact, Jesus labored so much that John says about Him at the close of his Gospel, "And there are also many other things that Jesus did, which, if every one of them were written down, I suppose not even the world itself could contain the books that would be written" (John 21:25). At times, the labor of Jesus developed into struggles. With each struggle, Jesus gained strength—strength which He can grant us. Jesus came through victorious in every struggle He faced!

In your journey, you can rely on the strength of Jesus to help you do all things needed to reach your weight loss goal. Losing weight requires intensive labor. If you thought we had discovered an easy, quick way to lose weight and keep it off, you must feel very disappointed. But if a little bit of work doesn't scare you, then we have some good news for you: you can do it!

Not only does losing weight require intensive labor, it can also present struggles. Once you reach your weight loss goal, the labor and struggles do not cease. One of the mistakes people make hinges on the false idea that once they reach that magic number, they can stop eating healthy and quit exercising.

Finally, see your journey as a spiritual one. Losing weight transforms your body into a living temple indwelt by the Spirit of God, operating at optimum efficiency for His glory! Just like Paul, you can say, "I am able to do all things through Him who strengthens me."

TAMMY'S TIDBITS

Our bodies serve as the living temples of God; and by exercising, we will have healthier living temples to serve our living God.

WEEK 5: DAY 6

Memory Verse: "I am able to do all things through him who strengthens me" (Phil. 4:13).

Challenge: Each day this week, take the stairs instead of the elevator for as many floors as possible without over-exertion.

Focus: Benefits of Friends

NATHAN'S NOTIONS

In today's devotion, we will consider a verse that occurs before our memory verse but helps set the context for Paul's bold statement. "I rejoiced in the Lord greatly because once again you renewed your care for me. You were, in fact, concerned about me but lacked the opportunity to show it" (Phil. 4:10). Paul experienced great joy in thinking about the loving care the Christians at Philippi bestowed upon him through financial support. After his love to his Lord Jesus, his love for the church at Philippi ranked second. His letter to them showed a deeper connection than he had with other churches. Paul rejoiced in the offering they made to him as proof of their love.

We all need help from time to time for many things, and losing weight is no exception. Friends can help us to come up with innovative ways to stay focused on our *Imagine Not as Much* journey. When you get stuck, think of the help you can receive from those in the support group.

As we develop as a group, let's hang on to the joy that comes from meeting together. Let's make a point to help each other every week. Spend time this week praying for those in your group. Spend time thanking God that He has brought them into your life.

Many people in the group stand ready and willing to show their love. Make it a point to let others know what you need to succeed. Give people an opportunity to get to know you and to help you along your journey. Look at it this way—you will purposely give someone an opportunity to show the love of Jesus in a practical way. No greater joy exists than that of serving our Lord; and when you open yourself to let others assist, you give them a chance at that joy.

TAMMY'S TIDBITS

If you do not have a church family, we encourage you to find one soon. You can start with the church hosting your Imagine Not as Much experience. If you already have a church family, make a point to invite an unchurched person to join you this week for worship.

WEEK 5: DAY 7

Memory Verse: "I am able to do all things through him who strengthens me" (Phil. 4:13).

Challenge: Each day this week, take the stairs instead of the elevator for as many floors as possible without over-exertion.

Challenge Carryover: Continue to take the stairs more often than you once did. You may not have the ability to take them every week because of sickness, tiredness, or soreness, and that's okay. Just try to take them at least once a week. You might gain such a physical benefit from doing so that you will want to take the stairs every day. If that's the case, then go for it!

Focus: Nutritional Fitness

NATHAN'S NOTIONS

Today's devotional will deal with the verses that immediately precede our memory verse. They tell us the secret that Paul found—contentment.

In our focus today on nutritional fitness, we bear in mind that temptation comes as we try to lose weight. One way to beat temptation resides in contentment. When we control our desires, we truly have the ability to do all things through Jesus.

We can learn contentment. Paul learned to experience it when in abundance and in poverty by trusting in the Savior. We can do the same. When we trust in Jesus to take care of our needs, we trust that He loves us and cares for us.

Now, some practical things that I do to maintain contentment in the two extremes of "whether well fed or hungry, whether in abundance or in need" (Phil. 4:12b). For the first, at buffets and church dinners, I practice "two plus one plus one then done," placing four servings on my plate: two vegetables, one starch, and one protein. At sit-down restaurants, I cut the serving in half and place it in a to-go box. For the second extreme, I intentionally eat healthy food six times a day to curb my hunger.

Think about how you will handle nutritional fitness for your eating extremes. Find a plan that works for you and brings you contentment. You can do it if you only *Imagine*!

TAMMY'S TIDBITS

Mindfully eat and enjoy the taste of your healthy food to reach contentment. Slow down; put your fork down; chew thoroughly; and don't take another bite until you cleanse your palate.

SECOND FOCUS: PHYSICAL FITNESS

"A thief comes only to steal and kill and destroy. I have come so that they may have life and have it in abundance" (John 10:10).

WEEK 6: ANAEROBIC EXERCISE

Another type of physical activity—anaerobic—builds muscle and stamina without taxing the lungs and heart. Some anaerobic activity may increase the heart rate and the breathing capacity, but for only a short period of time. Anaerobic activity focuses on strength-training.

Refer to the list of anaerobic activities below. Use the same process of circles and strikes.

TYPES OF ANAEROBIC ACTIVITIES

- Rowing
- Push-ups
- Pull-ups / Chin-ups
- Isometrics
- Sit-ups
- Weight Training
- Interval Training
- Sprints
- Tug of War
- Jumping Rope
- Climbing hills or stairs
- Squats
- Planking
- Yoga
- Tai Chi
- Pilates

We have included three routines for free weights, timed for sixty minutes, forty-five minutes, and thirty minutes. See below a description of the sixty-minute free weights routine.

BASIC WEIGHT-LIFTING INFORMATION

- You will need to use different size dumbbells, depending upon the exercise. Keep in mind two general rules of thumb: If you can lift the weight sixteen times easily, go heavier. If you cannot lift the weight eight times, go lighter.

- Practice proper form to avoid injury. We will explain this in the description of each exercise.

- When possible, exercise with a friend, in case of accidents or injuries.

- Listen to your body. If it hurts, stop.

- Recognize the difference between soreness from effective weight lifting and pain from improper weightlifting.

- The numbers we have included beside each exercise indicate repetitions (reps)—the number of times you will perform that particular movement.

- For floor exercises, use a mat. Nathan also has to use a pillow to support his back, and you may need to also.

DESCRIPTION OF EXERCISES AND MUSCLE GROUPS

- **Leg Raises (three ways): Abdominal**

This requires a bed or other raised soft surface, like an ottoman.

Lie on your back with your hands behind your head. Start with your legs resting comfortably over the side of the bed (or other surface). Raise them until they reach the horizontal position; then lower them. Repeat.

Start with your legs raised in the air. Lower them to the surface; then raise them again. Repeat.

Start with your legs raised in the air. Cross them four times. Lower them to a horizontal position, and cross them four times. Repeat.

- **Squats: Quadriceps**

Hold a dumbbell in each hand, palms facing inward. Stand with your feet about shoulder-width apart. Without going past perpendicular, bend your knees as low as you can while keeping your back straight. Return to a standing position. Repeat.

- **Lunges: Quadriceps**

Using dumbbell weights challenging yet comfortable for you, hold them in each hand, palms facing inward. Stand with your feet about shoulder-width apart. Move one leg forward, bending the opposite knee. Return to starting position, and repeat with the other leg. Repeat.

- **Hamstring presses: Hamstrings**

Get on the floor on all fours. Raise a straightened leg behind you, until it reaches a horizontal position. Curl the leg into your body, then back to a horizontal position. Repeat. Complete all the reps before switching to the other leg.

- **Kneeling butt-busters: Butt**

Assume the all-fours position. Bring one knee slightly off the floor. Move your leg upward, keeping it bent, as high as you can. Repeat. Complete all reps before switching to the other leg.

- **Outer leg lifts: Outer thighs**

Lie on the floor on your side. Raise the top leg up as high as you can without pain or injury. Lower until almost, but not quite, touching the other foot and leg. Repeat. Complete all reps before switching legs.

- **Inner leg lifts: Inner thighs**

Lie on the floor on your side. Bend the knee of the top leg with your foot on the floor. Now raise the lower leg as high as you can; then lower until almost, but not quite, touching the floor. Repeat. Complete all reps before switching legs.

- **Calf raises: Calves**

Stand with your feet about shoulder-width apart, holding two dumbbells. Stand on your tiptoes for a count of two; then lower to the floor. Repeat. For a more strenuous version, place your toes on a board, or use the stairs.

- **Back stretches: Back**

Lie on the floor on your stomach. Extend one arm, and raise the opposite leg. Hold while counting to five. Repeat with the other arm and alternate leg. Repeat.

- **Overhead back presses: Back**

Lie on the floor on your back. Take two dumbbells, and hold them at your chest with palms facing each other for the starting position. Raise them over your head, then behind your head almost touching the floor, keeping your arms relatively straight. Raise them straight up to complete the rep. Repeat.

- **Bench presses: Chest**

Lie on the floor on your back. Hold two dumbbells with palms facing forward, arms to the side at a ninety-degree angle to the floor. Extend your arms; then lower them. Repeat.

- **Butterflies: Chest**

Lie on the floor on your back. Hold two dumbbells with palms facing upward, arms extended and almost touching the floor. With arms extended but slightly bent, raise the dumbbells overhead till they touch. Lower. Repeat.

- **Vertical shoulder raises: Shoulders**

Stand with feet about shoulder-width apart. Hold two dumbbells with palms facing forward, arms at a ninety-degree angle and the weights just above the shoulders. Push straight up; then lower. Repeat.

- **Horizontal shoulder raises: Shoulders**

Stand with feet about shoulder-width apart. Hold two dumbbells with palms facing inward, arms hanging down straight in front of you. Lift the weights with arms relatively straight until they reach a ninety-degree angle; lower. Then move the weights to your sides. Lift them again, keeping arms relatively straight, until you reach a ninety-degree angle. Return to the starting position of palms facing inward. Repeat. This exercise utilizes the muscles involved in lifting the weights horizontally in front of you and on both sides.

- **Curls: Biceps**

Stand with feet about shoulder-width apart. Hold two dumbbells at your side near your thighs with palms facing forward. Curl the arm, until reaching just past a ninety-degree angle; then lower. Repeat. Make sure to use your arms only, and do not sway to gain leverage. Swaying will decrease the effectiveness of the exercise for your biceps and may injure your back.

- **Hammer curls: Biceps**

Stand with feet about shoulder-width apart. Hold two dumbbells at your side near your thighs with palms facing inward. Perform the movements for the curl. Repeat.

- **Triceps overhead: Triceps**

Stand with feet about shoulder-width apart. Hold two dumbbells with palms facing inward, arms over your head, with weights behind your head resting on your shoulders. Raise your arms over your head; then lower to behind your head. Repeat.

- **Triceps—one arm: Triceps**

Use the surface that aided with your leg raises in the first exercise. Kneel on the surface with one knee. With the opposite arm of bended knee, hold one dumbbell with palm facing inward and arm dangling. Raise the weight with a straight arm behind you until you reach a ninety-degree angle. Bend your arm at the elbow, pulling the weight to your side; extend again; then lower your arm to a dangling position. Repeat. Switch your kneeling position to exercise opposite arm.

- **Crunches three ways: Abdominal**

Lie on the floor on your back.

Place your arms over your chest. Raise your back off the floor, using your abdominal muscles. Hold for a count of one; then lower. Repeat.

Place your hands behind your head. As your raise your back, twist to one side. Hold for a count of one; then lower. Repeat.

Duplicate previous crunch with an opposite side twist. Repeat.

FREE WEIGHTS FOR SIXTY MINUTES

1. Leg raises @16 three ways
2. Squats @12
3. Lunges @12
4. Hamstring presses @12 by two legs
5. Kneeling butt busters @12 by two legs
6. Outer leg lifts @12 by two legs
7. Inner leg lifts @12 by two legs
8. Calf raises @12
9. Back stretches @12 by two legs
10. Overhead back presses @12
11. Bench presses @16
12. Butterflies @16
13. Vertical shoulder presses @16
14. Horizontal shoulder presses @8
15. Curls @16
16. Hammer Curls @16
17. Triceps overhead @16
18. Triceps one arm @16
19. Crunches @16 three ways

FREE WEIGHTS FOR FORTY-FIVE MINUTES

1. Leg raises @12 three ways
2. Squats @9
3. Lunges @9
4. Hamstring presses @9 by two legs
5. Kneeling butt busters @9 by two legs
6. Outer leg lifts @9 by two legs
7. Inner leg lifts @9 by two legs
8. Calf raises @9
9. Back stretches @9 by two legs
10. Overhead back presses @9
11. Bench presses @12
12. Butterflies @12
13. Vertical shoulder press @12
14. Horizontal shoulder press @6
15. Curls @12
16. Hammer curls @12
17. Triceps overhead @12
18. Triceps one arm @12
19. Crunches @12 three ways

FREE WEIGHTS FOR THIRTY MINUTES

1.	Leg raises @8 three ways	10.	Overhead back presses @6
2.	Squats @6	11.	Bench presses @8
3.	Lunges @6	12.	Butterflies @8
4.	Hamstring presses @6 by two legs	13.	Vertical shoulder press @8
5.	Kneeling butt busters @6 by two legs	14.	Horizontal shoulder press @4
6.	Outer leg lifts @6 by two legs	15.	Curls @8
7.	Inner leg lifts @6 by two legs	16.	Hammer curls @8
8.	Calf raises @6	17.	Triceps overhead @8
9.	Back stretches @6 by two legs	18.	Triceps one arm @8
		19.	Crunches @8 three ways

Other anaerobic exercises include planking, yoga, Tai Chi, Pilates, etc. As with nutritional fitness, the first few weeks you will practice a lot of experimentation. With both the aerobic and anaerobic activities, switch up the exercises and routines after eight to thirteen weeks. Our bodies get used to the routines, and the exercises lose their effectiveness. When we make changes, it works the muscles differently, making them work harder. We encourage you to experiment because you might find exercises you enjoy! Get moving. Just start! You can do it, and an Imaginator will help you each step of the way.

Tammy felt reluctant to try strength training. Nathan had done various forms over the years. From the sounds he made during his workouts, it did not sound fun. And Tammy remained unconvinced of its benefits.

Previously, you learned to do only exercises that you enjoy because you will do them more consistently and frequently. However, like Tammy, you may face reluctance to begin strength-training.

Tammy began a routine from a book that promoted eight minutes of weightlifting each day for six days and one day of rest over a four-week period. It worked different muscle groups each day. Tammy did not find those twenty-eight days easy; and most days, she did not like anything about it.

By the end of the twenty-eight days, she could see the results. The book had encouraged her to measure her neck, arms, chest, waist, and legs at the beginning and to measure those same areas at the end. She found that while she may not have lost as much weight during that period as she would have liked, she did lose up to an inch and a half in all areas!

That alone motivated her to continue. Strength-training still has not made it to her all-time favorite list, and she won't compete in any body-building events. However, she has found that strength training remains essential to maintaining her weight.

WEEK 6: DAY 1

Memory Verse: "A thief comes only to steal and kill and destroy. I have come so that they may have life and have it in abundance" (John 10:10).

Challenge: This week, increase your level of movement in creative ways in your normal activities. Examples include doing squats while cooking, walking in place while watching TV, or doing leg lefts while reading, etc.

Focus: Physical Fitness

NATHAN'S NOTIONS

In today's devotion time, we will look at the beginning of our memory verse. We know from the context that Jesus refers to Satan as the thief. The meaning stands in direct contrast to what Jesus offers to those who follow Him. Satan has developed three skills of theft, murder, and destruction.

Satan tries to steal our joy when he convinces us that we cannot enjoy all the good food God has provided and when we think about the short-term discomfort we feel while exercising. We combat this by remembering that God wants us to enjoy life to the fullest with a healthy, fit body.

Satan tries to kill our motivation by reminding us of our past failures and trying to convince us we will not do better now. He fills us with guilt in the present with every mistake, and he makes us think the future task ahead demands too much time and energy. We combat his efforts by reminding ourselves that God has forgiven us of our past; we ask for and receive God's forgiveness in the present; and we accept that we will work hard in the future to achieve what we want.

Satan tries to destroy our hope when he takes away our joy and kills our motivation. We lose hope that we will ever lose weight or that we will ever maintain a healthy body. Do not let him steal your joy of physical and nutritional fitness. Do not let him kill your motivation. Celebrate each victory knowing that you have taken the right steps to achieve a healthy body. Do not let him destroy your hope. "Because the one who is in you is greater than the one who is in the world" (1 John 4:4b).

TAMMY'S TIDBITS

Get creative during the day. Do leg lifts while standing still. Park farther away from the front door. If at work, take a ten-minute break to walk around. If at home, put dumbbells on the kitchen counter; instead of grabbing an unhealthy snack, grab the weights, and do a few reps!

WEEK 6: DAY 2

Memory Verse: "A thief comes only to steal and kill and destroy. I have come so that they may have life and have it in abundance" (John 10:10).

Challenge: This week, increase your level of movement in creative ways in your normal activities.

Focus: Benefits of Water

NATHAN'S NOTIONS

As stated yesterday, the purpose of the thief consists of theft, murder, and destruction. The purpose of Jesus' coming embodies the antithesis of the thief. Jesus has come to give instead of steal, to give life instead of murder, and to give life in abundance instead of destruction.

Today's devotional will not only consider the words of Jesus but also the benefits of water. Drinking sufficient amounts of water keeps us hydrated the entire day and acts as a lubricant for our bodies.[24] If you have stiffness in your joints or have trouble moving, try drinking at least sixty-four ounces of water a day.

The scriptural focus of today's devotion centers on the words of Jesus in our memory verse: "I have come so that they may have." Jesus' Divine authority rests in the fact that He came at just the right time. "When the time came to completion, God sent his Son, born of a woman, born under the law" (Gal. 4:4). Jesus came at the time prescribed by the Father, under the law. Jesus' Divine authority rests in His life upon the earth. Everything about Jesus clearly showed His Divine authority.

Jesus came with a mission of Divine love. Jesus willingly gave up the riches of Heaven to live among us and to die for us. His love superseded His own comfort, position in Heaven, and life.

TAMMY'S TIDBITS

Many fitness centers that have indoor pools offer water aerobics. Maybe you would enjoy this exercise. Water exercises in the summer could include swimming, rowing, canoeing, paddle boating, and fishing.

---

24 Reynolds, *Bod4God*, 135.

WEEK 6: DAY 3

Memory Verse: "A thief comes only to steal and kill and destroy. I have come so that they may have life and have it in abundance" (John 10:10).

Challenge: This week, increase your level of movement in creative ways in your normal activities.

Focus: Motivational Fitness

NATHAN'S NOTIONS

Today's and tomorrow's devotions will focus on the word "life" that Jesus used in John 10:10, which translates the Greek word *zoen*.[25] This word means several things.

This word "life" stands for spiritual life that only Jesus can bestow. He said, "I am the way, the truth, and the life. No one comes to the Father except through me" (John 14:6). As we begin a personal relationship with Jesus by inviting Him into our hearts through prayer, we discover the only way to experience spiritual life.

Zoen assures one of salvation from death. This life that we possess because of our relationship with Jesus brings with it the defeat of death (1 Cor. 15:54-57).

Zoen also represents a new and Divine principle. Because of *zoen*, life has a purpose, a design, and a future all wrapped up in a personal relationship with Jesus.

In today's focus of motivational fitness, remember that God the Father loves you so much that He provided *zoen* through His Son Jesus. God wants you to experience the best in life as you embrace a spiritual life with Him, rejoice in salvation from death, and celebrate His new and Divine principle. Once you reach your weight loss goal, you will feel better, have the ability to do more for your Lord, and help others discover *zoen* by inviting them on the journey with you!

TAMMY'S TIDBITS

By now, you more than likely feel better. Give yourself a pat on the back, and celebrate your accomplishment! Let this feeling of accomplishment encourage you and motivate you. Right now, do some sort of activity for a couple of minutes: stretch; walk around the house; do a few crunches; or lift some light weights.

---

25 Rudolf Bultmann, "The Concept of Life in the N.T.," *Theological Dictionary of the New Testament* (Grand Rapids: Wm. B. Eerdmans Publishing Company, 1964), 2:861-875.

WEEK 6: DAY 4

Memory Verse: "A thief comes only to steal and kill and destroy. I have come so that they may have life and have it in abundance" (John 10:10).

Challenge: This week, increase your level of movement in creative ways in your normal activities.

Challenge Check-up: How have you done this week in finding creative ways to increase your level of movement? I know that some of the ways you may have tried seemed silly at the time, and that's okay. Every calorie burned counts, even the silly ones!

Focus: Benefits of Effective Time Management

NATHAN'S NOTIONS

Another Greek word for "life"—*bios*—means natural life, and thus follows a predictable path to decay and dissolution.[26] The word for "life" from our memory verse—*zoen*—stands different in that it progresses instead of decays. This spiritual life begins at the moment of salvation and continues to progress until fully realized in Heaven. "For now we see only a reflection as in a mirror, but then face to face. Now I know in part, but then I will know fully, as I am fully known" (1 Cor. 13:12).

Our *zoen* progresses at the rate we allow it. For some, the progression remains slow (Heb. 5:11-13). For others, the progression continues at a rapid pace, producing mature believers who embrace the lives God has called them to live. Regardless, *zoen* embodies progression instead of decay.

In this regard of progression, we see the importance of effective time management be-cause making time to spend with God will help you lose weight. When we make time for God, we can put everything else in perspective, including eating healthy and exercising regularly.

In reference to human life, *bios* begins at the moment of conception and continues until the heart stops beating. It has a beginning, and it has an end. Whereas in reference to human life, *zoen* begins the moment someone accepts Jesus Christ as Savior and never ends. This "life" has a beginning, but no end. *Bios* has a natural progression to decay and death—for some faster than others. *Zoen* has a natural progression of vitality and eternity—again, for some faster than others. The apostle John uses the Greek word *zoen* in John 10:10 (cf. John 11:25-26).

TAMMY'S TIDBITS

Think creatively with your time management. You can use this time as a great opportu-nity to experiment with different types of activities. Try bike riding, swimming, jumping rope, or hula hooping.

---

26 Bultmann, 2:851-854.

WEEK 6: DAY 5

Memory Verse: "A thief comes only to steal and kill and destroy. I have come so that they may have life and have it in abundance" (John 10:10).

Challenge: This week, increase your level of movement in creative ways in your normal activities.

Focus: Spiritual Fitness

NATHAN'S NOTIONS

In today's devotion time, we will begin to consider the words "and have it in abundance." Looking at the abundant life we have in Jesus will guide our thoughts for the remainder of this week. Today's focus draws attention to spiritual fitness.

Jesus gives us abundant life in that He sets our lives on their true course away from a life of destruction, misery, and spiritual death. We have meaning and possess a purpose when we know we face the right direction in life.

When Jesus gives us abundant life, He gives us the ability to exercise all the powers available to us. Whereas before we experienced only a portion of our capabilities, through Jesus, we can make use of all of them.

Jesus' gift of abundant life brings joy in our hearts. Without Jesus, we tend to focus on the negative and wallow in pity. With the touch of Jesus, we respond to circumstances differently.

Jesus' gift of abundant life allows us to have supremacy over all things in life. Trying times abound when attempting to lose weight. You will make mistakes along the way. But nothing has the power to overwhelm you and take away your *zoen*. You have supremacy over getting knocked down. Keep trusting in the Lord Jesus to help you reach your goal and maintain spiritual fitness. You will overcome the evil one with the abundant life!

TAMMY'S TIDBITS

We can also think creatively in making time for our spiritual fitness by talking with God on our drive to work. I use that time to pray for my friends and family and other special needs or ministries.

WEEK 6: DAY 6

Memory Verse: "A thief comes only to steal and kill and destroy. I have come so that they may have life and have it in abundance" (John 10:10).

Challenge: This week, increase your level of movement in creative ways in your normal activities.

Focus: Benefits of Friends

NATHAN'S NOTIONS

In today's devotion, we will look at some more meanings of life in abundance and how they help us to live out the truth of our faith among others.

Jesus' gift of abundant life kindles an enthusiasm for doing good. Abundant life in Jesus creates a spark in our hearts to want to try to live our lives for His glory.

Jesus' gift of abundant life also allows us to experience deeper feelings toward others. We begin to see our lives as instruments through which the love of Christ can flow. Many people in our community struggle with losing weight. Each one of us who have gone through this journey can work together to help others also achieve success in reaching and maintaining a healthy weight. As our eyes become open to the people around us needing the Savior's touch and our feelings deepen with the abundant life of Jesus, we can help many discover hope.

Jesus' gift of abundant life enlarges our sphere of things. We no longer consider the events that happen around us as the extent of our existence; rather, we open ourselves to expansion as Jesus moves within our hearts. With abundant life in Jesus, we have the privilege and joy of thinking about making an impact beyond what we currently know. Each day awaits as an adventure in serving God.

TAMMY'S TIDBITS

A creative way to invite friends to exercise could involve a competition. Find someone who shares similar interests to decide what activity, goal, and stakes. Don't forget to have fun!

WEEK 6: DAY 7

Memory Verse: "A thief comes only to steal and kill and destroy. I have come so that they may have life and have it in abundance."

Challenge: This week, increase your level of movement in creative ways in your normal activities.

Challenge Carryover: As you continue this practice, keep making it fun and creative. You can continue doing the things that have worked and just leave yourself open to new ideas as they pop into your head. Before too long, your old couch potato self will turn into a calorie-burning machine.

Focus: Nutritional Fitness

NATHAN'S NOTIONS

Let's look at the remaining meanings of life in abundance as it relates to nutritional fitness. The abundant life offers more energy. When we have a desire to do something worthwhile, it increases our levels of energy. Living in abundance means that we look forward to each new day in the presence of Jesus because we know He has something exciting in store for us.

The abundant life offers more stamina. When we spend time with the Lord, we have the energy to do what it takes to complete a task that He has placed on our hearts. This also applies to the food we eat. When we eat healthy foods, they fuel our bodies, giving us more stamina to do the work Christ has called us to do.

The abundant life keeps our minds focused on the transforming truths of God. We set our minds on things that make a difference in our lives, instead of the base, carnal things of the earth.

Let's think about living our lives for the glory of God instead of satisfying our fleshly desires. Let's dwell on having a healthy body in which to more effectively serve the Lord. Let's choose actions that will help us to honor God in what we eat and drink and how we use our bodies. Your future appears bright with abundant life as a person who serves God to the best of their ability—with a healthy and fit body!

TAMMY'S TIDBITS

Try to think creatively with your food. Try some spaghetti squash or eggplant, or treat yourself to an exotic fruit or vegetable. Google "healthy recipes" and check out new ideas. Share with your group what new food you tried and your newly discovered recipes.

THIRD FOCUS: MOTIVATIONAL FITNESS

"And so, after waiting patiently, Abraham obtained the promise" (Heb. 6:15).

WEEK 7: MOTIVATION

We have spent the last several weeks discussing the importance of nutritional and physical fitness for effective weight loss. We will spend the next three weeks focusing on another important aspect of weight loss: engaging your mind.

Unless you make up your mind that you will lose weight, you will not succeed. Change your way of thinking. Don't think of *Imagine Not as Much* just as a weight loss journey; think of it also as a healthy lifestyle journey because you do not simply want to lose weight; you want to achieve and maintain a healthier lifestyle.

No one likes change. We get used to the way we do things, and change alters our lives. Many times, we see an alteration in a negative light on how it impacts us. Let's change our outlook on change and view it as perseverance, steadfastness, and endurance—all aspects needed for successful weight loss.

Nathan imagined a couple of things when he lost weight and achieved his goal. He imagined tying his tennis shoes without his face turning red and getting out of breath. He also imagined saying, "I would love to" when his grandchildren asked him to play.

These things helped to motivate him to get started and stay strong in his conviction to lose weight. He knew lots of temptations awaited him, but he determined to take on the challenges needed to achieve his goal. Motivational fitness conveys, "I can do it, and I will do it, period."

We both noticed early in our weight loss journeys how much better we felt. We did not feel as lethargic in the afternoons. We noticed we could take the stairs without our knees hurting or feeling completely winded at the top. Indigestion improved dramatically, and we felt more energetic in doing simple things.

We also discovered that if we ate unhealthily, the icky feeling that we experienced as a part of our everyday lives before we began losing weight returned, and we did not like that! Feeling better comprises a strong motivator to lose weight. Some have discovered a reduction or elimination of medication due to their Imagine Not as Much experience and have found the desire to maintain their medicinal changes as a strong motivation to continue losing weight and to keep it off!

Tammy's clothes became looser. She, of course, noticed this before other people did. But once she had to buy a size smaller clothes, she liked it. She felt like a pretender the first time she shopped in the Misses part of the department store.

Tammy does not imagine as well as Nathan. But fitting into smaller sizes provided a strong motivation for her. It encouraged her to continue. Tammy had to fight the thoughts, "I look okay at my current size. I look so much better than I did; let's just stop." Here's the truth. She had not obtained a healthy weight. She imagined the scale saying her goal weight, and she wanted to fight until she got there. A fight truly describes the struggle.

The clothes you wear can serve as great motivation. As you lose weight, they will become looser. You will need to buy a smaller size or a smaller belt. Give away your old clothes as they get too big. This will motivate you as you won't have them as a crutch if you gain weight. It proves easier and more fun to buy clothes when you reach a smaller size than when you have to because your size increases!

How do you imagine your life when you meet you weight goal? Record your answer:

_____

_____

_____

_____

_____

Imagine your celebration when you meet your goal weight. A recent conversation Tammy had with a co-worker illustrates this point. Tammy's wedding rings had become very loose since she lost weight. She planned on celebrating her goal weight by having the rings re-sized. Her friend at work said, "Why don't you go ahead and have them sized now if you have only five pounds left?" Nathan promised Tammy that when she met her goal weight, she could have the rings re-sized as her reward. Yes, she could have the rings sized sooner—five pounds would not make that much of a difference. It made a difference to Tammy, though, and helped her to lose those last five pounds.

Imagine how you will celebrate once you make your goal. Your celebration may include a trip for you and someone special, buying yourself an item of jewelry that you have had your eye on, or purchasing something special for which you have to save money to buy. Your celebration may contain food as you enjoy a healthy meal with someone you love. You could also celebrate by donating or selling your old ill-fitting clothes or having the ones you really enjoy altered to fit your new body. You could also celebrate by posting before and after pictures of yourself on social media after you reach your goal. Whatever you can imagine as a way to commemorate your success determines your personal celebration! What will you do?

Record your celebration here:

_____

_____

_____

_____

_____

The mind: your most powerful weight loss tool. Without the power of your mind, you cannot follow through with nutritional fitness or physical fitness. With the power of your mind, you can achieve both. Your weight-loss journey will not work unless you put your mind to it!

WEEK 7: DAY 1

Memory Verse: "And so, after waiting patiently, Abraham obtained the promise" (Heb. 6:15).

Challenge: This week, decide that you will reach your weight-loss goal.

Focus: Motivational Fitness

NATHAN'S NOTIONS

Our memory verse this week focuses on Abraham. The context of the verse reminds us not only of the Abraham in history but also of the descendants of Abraham. The assurances made to Abraham about obtaining the promise have continued in a spiritual sense throughout Christianity, confirmed by the death of Jesus on the cross of Calvary and sealed by His resurrection from the dead and ascension into Heaven. Paul writes, "For every one of God's promises is 'Yes' in him. Therefore, through him we also say 'Amen' to the glory of God" (2 Cor. 1:20). God cares about us, and He wants the best for us, including the healthiest life we can live. We have the example of Abraham before us that the promise will come true.

In order to lose weight effectively and keep it off, we must first of all believe that we can do it! Sometimes getting started seems hard because we may say discouraging things to ourselves like, "Why try *Imagine Not as Much*? Nothing you have tried has worked before." Or, "I know you won't stick with it. You may do good for a couple of weeks or maybe a couple of months, but then you will just gain all the weight back." I said the very same things to myself when I began this journey. I put all of those negative thoughts behind me and believed in myself, and that made a huge difference.

Abraham represents a great example of clinging to the promise of God, even though he could not see immediate results. Take from this biblical example, and trust that you will reach your goal. You will become a healthier version of you. You will *Imagine Not as Much*!

TAMMY'S TIDBITS

Determine to stick with it. Make up your mind that you **WILL** lose weight.

WEEK 7: DAY 2

Memory Verse: "And so, after waiting patiently, Abraham obtained the promise" (Heb. 6:15).

Challenge: This week, decide that you will reach your weight loss goal.

Focus: Benefits of Water

NATHAN'S NOTIONS

Our memory verse this week starts with two simple words from the Greek New Testament: *kai*,[27] *houto*,[28] "and so." Because of their simplicity and common occurrence, we may gloss over them, believing the other words carry more weight in meaning. But these two simple words possess power. Every time these words occur together in Scripture, they always refer to a previous statement. Two examples of their occurrence appear in the Greek New Testament in Acts 7:8 and Acts 28:14. To fully understand the meaning of "and so," we must know what immediately precedes them in our memory verse. Hebrews 6:13-14 reads, "For when God made a promise to Abraham, since he had no one greater to swear by, he swore by himself: **I will indeed bless you, and I will greatly multiply you.**"

God made a solemn vow to Abraham that He would bless and multiply him. It did not matter that Abraham had no land and no children or how God planned to carry out His promise. God said it, and Abraham believed it. The absolute promise of an unfailing God served as the basis for his "and so." What defines your "and so?" Do you confidently believe that God cares for you and wants the best for you? Do you believe that He has provided everything you need to live a healthy life? We have everything we need at our disposal to lead a healthy life and to achieve a healthy weight.

Take water, for example. It exists in abundant supply, and it flows freely from the tap or the water fountain! Even if you have to pay for it, you can buy it cheaply in gallon jugs. God has provided the greatest hydration liquid ever, but many of us pass it up for something that has more flavor and calories. Today, choose to act upon your belief that God loves you and wants the best for you. Today, get motivated and live out your "and so!"

TAMMY'S TIDBITS

Water lets our bodies know if we crave hunger or thirst. When you think you experience hunger, take a drink of water. If the hunger pang passes, then you quenched your thirst.

---

27 Thayer, 315-317.
28 Ibid, 468-469.

WEEK 7: DAY 3

Memory Verse: "And so, after waiting patiently, Abraham obtained the promise" (Heb. 6:15).

Challenge: This week, decide that you will reach your weight-loss goal.

Focus: Spiritual Fitness

NATHAN'S NOTIONS

Let's look at the last three words of our memory verse: "obtained the promise." Abraham obtained the promise of God after a time of waiting patiently. God promised Abraham, **"I will indeed bless you, and I will greatly multiply you"** (Heb. 6:14). We have the same promise. He waits for us to act upon His promise of blessing and multiplying. We act upon it by believing and inviting into our hearts God's Son and submitting to Him as Lord.

We experience God's blessings when we obey Him. When we follow the directions God gives, we discover the blessings of life—the opportunity to demonstrate to others what it means to live in true fellowship with God with a joyful heart and a thankful spirit. They, in turn, will want to know more, and thus, we multiply as others invite Jesus into their hearts and submit to Him as Lord.

Sometimes, as overweight people, we feel guilty about how we have treated our bodies. We know that we should eat healthier; we know we should exercise more. Instead of doing something to change, we give up and resign ourselves to living in guilt.

We rationalize our guilt over not losing weight. We care more about what we eat and enjoying leisure time than we care about honoring God with our bodies or how our testimonies negatively affect others. Tammy and I want you to know that you can obtain the promise of a blessed life. You can make the choice to live your life in a healthy manner to glorify God. Once you begin to lose weight and people notice, you will stay motivated to continue until you have "obtained the promise."

TAMMY'S TIDBITS

Guilt can keep us from a healthy relationship with the Lord. Ask the Lord to forgive you, and then do one more thing: forgive yourself. Once God has forgiven you and you have forgiven yourself, then you can move on and "obtain the promise."

WEEK 7: DAY 4

Memory Verse: "And so, after waiting patiently, Abraham obtained the promise" (Heb. 6:15).

Challenge: This week, decide that you will reach your weight loss goal.

Challenge Check-up: Record your weight-loss goal. Determine that no matter the obstacles and no matter how difficult it seems, you will reach your goal. Decide this simple truth in your heart, mind, and spirit, and your body will follow suit.

Focus: Benefits of Effective Time Management

NATHAN'S NOTIONS

Let's look at three words in English that translate to only one word in Greek: "after waiting patiently," which translates, *macrothumesas*.[29] This word can also translate as "being long-suffering" or "after he had patiently endured." These words connect to similar words in Hebrews 6:12, which reads, "So that you won't become lazy but will be imitators of those who inherit the promises through faith and perseverance." When we patiently wait for something to happen, we can lose sight of what we do. We live in such a fast-paced society today that we want immediate results. That's why weight-loss programs that promise ten pounds lost in seven days gain popularity. However, the results do not last, and most people gain back more weight than they lost.

In week one, we asked you to set a target weight for thirteen weeks based upon losing one to two pounds a week. We know that one pound may represent an insignificant amount. However, losing between half-a-pound and two pounds a week constitutes healthy weight loss, and it takes time. The significance arises when you consider its cumulative, permanent results. What you learn in this journey will help keep the weight off once you lose it. But you have to wait patiently. From Hebrews 6:12, we learn that perseverance or waiting patiently does not constitute laziness. It takes a committed person to wait patiently while your body changes until you begin to see lasting results. Setting specific goals forms the basis for long-term success. You have to have the final result clear in your mind.

You can cling to hope while waiting patiently for your goal to materialize. Faith precedes hope. Whereas faith *reveals* the possibility, hope *anticipates* the possibility. Spiritual diligence bears the fruit of hope. The sweet aroma of hope wafts from the perspiration of effort! Today, choose to have abundant hope as you wait patiently to obtain the promise!

TAMMY'S TIDBITS

Keep your goal in mind, and try breaking it down into smaller increments.

---

29 J. Horst, "*makrothumeo* and *makrothumia* in the New Testament" *Theological Dictionary of the New Testament* (Grand Rapids: Wm. B. Eerdmans Publishing Company,1967), 4:379-387.

WEEK 7: DAY 5

Memory Verse: "And so, after waiting patiently, Abraham obtained the promise" (Heb. 6:15).

Challenge: This week, decide that you will reach your weight-loss goal.

Focus: Nutritional Fitness

NATHAN'S NOTIONS

Let's look at the historical Abraham to determine why the writer of Hebrews chose him to illustrate faith and hope as sure anchors of the soul. When Abraham was seventy-five, God promised him that He would bless him and greatly multiply his descendants. Abraham waited patiently for the fulfillment of the Promise; and finally, after twenty-five years of anticipation, his wife, Sarah, gave birth to their son, Isaac. Then we come to chapter twenty-two in the book of Genesis, where God asks Abraham to sacrifice his son.

Genesis 22 unfolds the story that shows the true test of Abraham's faith. It shows that Abraham believed God and trusted Him, even in the midst of uncertainty. The test of our faith does not come when things make perfectly good sense. Our test of faith comes when we have to make a choice: "Do I believe what I can figure out on my own, or do I believe God?" Abraham chose to believe God. Even though God stayed his hand and spared Isaac, Abraham's willingness stayed firm in following God's leadership. Abraham's test of faith did not consist of sacrificing his son or not. It consisted of his belief that God would bring Isaac back to life, even though Abraham did not know how.

In the sternest test of Abraham's faith rested the most blessed manifestation of Divine favor. Your test of faith will occur when you hit a plateau and do not see any significant change. If you wait patiently, you will obtain the Promise, just as Abraham did. Today, choose to exercise your faith, and stay true to your new eating plan—not a short-term diet but a lifestyle change you can do for the rest of your life!

TAMMY'S TIDBITS

It may seem tempting to think it a sacrifice eating healthily as opposed to eating whatever you want, but like Abraham, giving of yourself constitutes the real sacrifice. Today, purposely choose a new, healthy alternative to a food that you love. For instance, Nathan loves Snickers. He has discovered a chocolate-covered granola bar serves as a healthier but delicious alternative.

WEEK 7: DAY 6

Memory Verse: "And so, after waiting patiently, Abraham obtained the promise" (Heb. 6:15).

Challenge: This week, decide that you will reach your weight-loss goal.

Focus: Benefits of Friends

NATHAN'S NOTIONS

There remains hope that we will attain our weight-loss goal when we put it into God's hands. Just as Abraham trusted in the promises of God and remained patiently waiting for Him to fulfill those promises, we can do the same. We can have hope while trying to lose weight by ourselves, but friends can help us along the journey by thinking of ideas for weight loss that we may never have considered. Those ideas can prevent us from drifting away. Even though we know what we need to do to lose weight, we can still get carried away with all the fads. Friends can help us stay focused on what truly works—eating less, eating healthier, and exercising more.

Friends can also help us in the storms that will arise through temptations by reminding us that if we will stay the course and do the right thing, we will receive a huge pay-off. We will obtain the promise!

Friends can become our biggest cheering section by helping us to see that our goal appears closer today than a week ago, or even just one day ago. When we have a lot of weight to lose, we can easily become discouraged. Friends remind us that our journey consists of a lifelong experience, not a quick fix solution or diet. This program represents a lifestyle change that will take time to develop. Friends will remind you that you have invested well in your time to make this change and to complete the journey, so one day you can say, "I obtained the promise!"

TAMMY'S TIDBITS

If you do not belong to an Imagine Not as Much group, think about starting one. You can begin by telling people that you need help losing weight, and they can assist you greatly by holding you accountable. If you have attended a group but dropped out, rejoin. The benefits you will experience will far outweigh any amount of embarrassment or guilt associated with your absence.

WEEK 7: DAY 7

Memory Verse: "And so, after waiting patiently, Abraham obtained the promise" (Heb. 6:15).

Challenge: This week, decide that you will reach your weight-loss goal.

Challenge Carryover: Each week as you weigh in, keep your weight-loss goal in mind. On the weeks that you lose weight, celebrate and vow to continue doing the things that work! On the weeks that you gain weight, try to pinpoint the reasons and vow to not repeat them again. Keep doing this each week until you reach your goal!

Focus: Physical Fitness

NATHAN'S NOTIONS

If you follow the eating plan that we suggest, you will lose weight. However, to maintain your weight-loss goal permanently, you must include physical fitness into your daily routine. Physical fitness helps your body more efficiently burn calories. If you stand ready to obtain the promise of effective and long-lasting weight loss, then you stand ready to achieve a healthier body. At first, you may experience soreness; but once your body gets used to moving and doing, the soreness will go away. Physical fitness certainly reminds us that we must wait patiently. It does not happen overnight; and at first, we might not notice a significant improvement to justify the effort. But just wait, patiently, and the effort will pay off.

I remember the first time I started weight-lifting. The person helping me told me two very important things: 1) you will not look like Arnold Schwarzenegger, and 2) you will experience soreness when you first start, but just stay with it. He spoke truth. After four weeks, my soreness began to wear off, and I felt like a new person! I had more energy, and I lost inches. I encourage you to stay with the principles you are learning. They will work; you will feel better; you will lose weight; and you will keep it off. This week, decide that you will reach your weight-loss goal. Let's finish this week's devotional by doing our memory verse just a little bit differently: "And so, after waiting patiently, (insert your name) obtained the promise." Won't it feel great when that statement rings true for you?

TAMMY'S TIDBITS

Add strength training to your exercise regimen to help with losing inches in addition to losing weight. Refer to week six for ideas.

THIRD FOCUS: MOTIVATIONAL FITNESS

"Whoever loves discipline loves knowledge, but one who hates correction is stupid" (Prov. 12:1).

WEEK 8: MENTAL ROADBLOCKS

We want to help you tap into the potential of imagination and the power of your mind. We want to share some things that they learned to help break through several mental roadblocks.

First mental roadblock: emotional eating. Imagine eating only when hungry. Emotional eating occurs with boredom, stress, sadness, feeling overwhelmed, or feeling happy. Identify the reason for eating. If not hungry, try to find other ways to deal with your emotional issues. Instead of eating, take a walk; read a book; distract yourself; find other ways to reward yourself; breathe deeply.

Identify times when you indulge in emotional eating. Record in the space below:

_____

_____

_____

_____

Second mental roadblock: addictive foods. Imagine eating only when you want to and not when you feel compelled to. Stay away from addictive foods, such as sweets and salty foods, as much as possible, especially in the beginning. Eat in moderation, and enjoy every bite, no matter what food you eat. Eat slowly; savor the flavor. Let's compare a bag of chips to a bag of apples for an example. You could probably eat an entire bag of chips in one sitting, whereas you could only finish two or three apples before having to stop.

List addictive foods for you. How do you plan on handling them?

_____

_____

_____

_____

Third mental roadblock: a house full of unhealthy foods. Imagine your house with only healthy food easily accessible. Purge your house of unhealthy foods. If you must have something tempting in your house, put it in a cabinet that you rarely use. Utilize the cabinet that you go to the most for your healthy choices. Entice your taste buds with healthy foods by putting them at eye level and in front of your cabinet or refrigerator.

What foods do you know you have to purge from your house?

_____

_____

_____

_____

_____

Fourth mental roadblock: planning ahead. Imagine what healthy eating looks like when you plan ahead to go to the grocery store, when you plan ahead for your daily eating, and when you plan ahead on eating out.

How will you plan ahead to go to the store?

_____

_____

_____

_____

_____

How will you plan ahead for your daily calorie intake?

_____

_____

_____

_____

How will you plan ahead when you eat out?

_____

_____

_____

_____

Fifth mental roadblock: plateaus. Imagine how you will conquer plateaus. Tammy encountered many plateaus. Each time, she reacted with anger. Although she worked hard, the number on the scale refused to move. Talk about frustration! Tammy got so angry, she did not want to quit or let the plateau get the best of her. So, she started "tweaking," really looking at the details, measuring each food serving, and adding dairy. The lesson she learned? Pay attention to details when in a plateau.

Little things add up quickly, like the extra calories from the coffee creamer or the mayo on the sandwich you had at lunch. Or while cooking, you taste everything twice to make sure it tastes good. Cutting those small steps could save up to five pounds in a year.

What do you consider a plateau?

_____

_____

_____

_____

What will you do about it when it happens?

_____

_____

_____

_____

Sixth mental roadblock: healthy eating saboteurs. Imagine how you will effectively handle saboteurs. You have those people who have made something special, and you *must* try it, but you know it has one thousand calories in one bite. These people will say, "Oh, come on, one bite's not going to kill you," or, "I made this just for you because I know you love it so much." Tammy learned a simple phrase that helps tremendously: "No, thank you, maybe later." This really works. She has not hurt any feelings and yet remained true to her "lifestyle change." Think of this program as a lifestyle change, not a diet.

Who constitutes the healthy eating saboteurs in your life, and when do they typically strike?

_____

_____

_____

_____

Seventh mental roadblock: feeling alone in your weight-loss journey. Imagine having people help you along the way. Accountability helps tremendously in effective weight loss.

Ask for help when temptations arise—like cookies in the breakroom that you want really badly. A good friend will know your dedication to this lifestyle change and support you. If you don't have that support, work at finding someone who will give it to you. You may find that someone in this group.

List the people to whom you will practice accountability:

_____

_____

_____

_____

Eighth mental roadblock: making mistakes. Imagine yourself recovering when you make an unhealthy food choice or do not make time to exercise one day. Forgive yourself. So what, you had a donut for breakfast. You can still eat a healthy lunch or dinner. We don't want you to deprive yourself. We just want you to obtain a healthy weight.

What steps will you take to recover from your mistakes?

_____

_____

_____

_____

WEEK 8: DAY 1

Memory Verse: "Whoever loves discipline loves knowledge, but one who hates correction is stupid" (Prov. 12:1).

Challenge: This week, forgive yourself for making mistakes. Refocus on what you need to do, and continue on to success.

Focus: Motivational Fitness

NATHAN'S NOTIONS

During our devotion time this week, we will look at our memory verse, along with several verses from the book of Proverbs. We will focus today on motivational fitness. When we get motivated to lose weight, we willingly do what it takes to accomplish the goal. We see instruction as necessary to reach our goal, and we learn to love the process, even when it seems difficult.

Some people have trouble getting motivated. They see encouragement as a negative, critical influence. The Scripture calls these people "stupid" or "brutish," but not ignorant. The difference between ignorance and stupidity lies in knowledge. An ignorant person does not know what to do; a stupid person knows what to do but refuses to do it. This week, we will look at "stupid" people. We will identify their characteristics, their paths of life, and their end result. Then we will look at the opposite.

A stupid person thinks only about the here and now in satisfying temporary, earthly pleasures. Proverbs 18:1 describes this person's characteristics when it says, "One who isolates himself pursues selfish desires; he rebels against all sound wisdom." Some satisfy their desires through drugs, alcohol, or unhealthy, shallow personal relationships. Still others look to eating unhealthy foods in enormous portions. The path of people addicted to satisfying their fleshly desires leads them to discover others who do the same. They rationalize that since others participate, it must be fine. Proverbs 23:20-21 warns us, "Don't associate with those who drink too much wine or with those who gorge themselves on meat. For the drunkard and the glutton will become poor, and grogginess will clothe them in rags." The one who thinks only of fulfilling their immediate desires will lament at the end of their life as their body shows extensive wear and tear. Don't follow the example of this type of stupid person. Imagine your body as a holy temple of God.

TAMMY'S TIDBITS

Stop the negative thinking. Instead, try to replace the negative thought with something positive.

WEEK 8: DAY 2

Memory Verse: "Whoever loves discipline loves knowledge, but one who hates correction is stupid" (Prov. 12:1).

Challenge: This week, forgive yourself for making mistakes. Refocus on what you need to do, and continue on to success.

Focus: Benefits of Water

NATHAN'S NOTIONS

A stupid person trusts in their pride. Proverbs 11:2a says about them, "When arrogance comes, disgrace follows." They believe they know the best course of action and feel confident in their decisions. Success makes one feel like there exists no need for instruction or correction. Proverbs 12:15a reminds us, "A fool's way is right in his own eyes."

The paths of prideful people seem like success stories. They achieve some recognition for a job well done and think that all they do resonates with what's right. They hate correction, balk at the idea of instruction, and try to convince others that their way offers the only way. Proverbs 29:23a tells us, "A person's pride will humble him."

Eventually, the pride of people will catch up to them. Humility lurks just around the corner. Prideful people do not believe truth when it contradicts something they have accepted as fact. For instance, if they have lived their entire lives without drinking water on a regular basis, they see no need to change because they have done fine up to this point. They refuse to accept the many proven benefits of drinking at least sixty-four ounces of water a day, including that it may help prevent asthma.[30]

Proverbs 16:18 puts it this way: "Pride comes before destruction, and an arrogant spirit before a fall." Eventually, pride will cause destruction in your life and a great fall. Don't let pride keep you stupid. Admit to God and others that you need help to lose weight, and you stand ready to receive whatever instruction or advice that will help. Put your pride down long enough to get help.

TAMMY'S TIDBITS

Most of the time, we don't drink water for the taste or lack thereof. If we can develop a taste to drink something unhealthy, we can also develop a taste to drink water. Don't let your pride get in the way for developing a taste for water!

---

30 Reynolds, *Bod4God*, 135.

WEEK 8: DAY 3

Memory Verse: "Whoever loves discipline loves knowledge, but one who hates correction is stupid" (Prov. 12:1).

Challenge: This week, forgive yourself for making mistakes. Refocus on what you need to do, and continue on to success.

Focus: Spiritual Fitness

NATHAN'S NOTIONS

A stupid person exemplifies slothfulness—having the idea that the least they can do in life, the better. The modern term "slacker" conveys the same term as "slothful" in Old Testament times. Proverbs 26:13-16 gives colorful commentary on those who practice slothfulness. It states, "The slacker says, 'There's a lion in the road—a lion in the public square!' A door turns on its hinges, and a slacker, on his bed. The slacker buries his hand in the bowl; he is too weary to bring it to his mouth. In his own eyes, a slacker is wiser than seven men who can answer sensibly."

Slackers see no benefit in changing anything in their routines because that means more work. As far as fitness goes, they remain comfortable sitting on their sofas eating unhealthy food while watching television. They hate correction because they want to remain exactly the same.

The journey of a slacker illustrates the popular notion of taking the path of least resistance. They do as little as they can for as long as they can. This remains true in physical activity and in spiritual activity. Slackers will make no effort at gaining knowledge through instruction in spiritual fitness and can expect poverty of spirit. They can expect the end result found in Proverbs 21:25, which tells us, "A slacker's craving will kill him because his hands refuse to work."

Healthy living benefits everything in our lives by improving our nutritional, physical, motivational, and spiritual fitness; but it takes hard work. If you follow the stupid example of the slacker, you will do nothing to improve your health and will eventually die due to complications resulting from your choices. Many diseases and ailments that cause premature death directly correspond to unhealthy eating habits and lack of physical activity. Don't die early. Live healthy; live long; and live for the Lord!

TAMMY'S TIDBITS

God loves us more than we can imagine and, out of that love, wants to spend time with us. Find some extra time for you and the Lord. He makes time for you; you can make time for Him.

WEEK 8: DAY 4

Memory Verse: "Whoever loves discipline loves knowledge, but one who hates correction is stupid."

Challenge: This week, forgive yourself for making mistakes. Refocus on what you need to do, and continue on to success.

Challenge Checkup: Have you made a mistake yet this week? If you haven't, you will. Do not let a mistake derail you from your goal of losing weight. One of the pitfalls of effective weight loss resides in the truth that once people mess up, they quit, thinking, "What's the use? I can't keep it up." Yes, you can. Forgive yourself first; then get back on track.

Focus: Benefits of Effective Time Management

NATHAN'S NOTIONS

In today's devotion, we will consider disciplined people. They freely forgo temporary enjoyment for the sake of a future benefit. They see the need in planning ahead and making provisions to reach their goals. They love discipline that leads to knowledge because it helps them meet their goals.

Disciplined people listen to instruction, even if it comes in the form of correction, because they realize the benefit. They understand the importance of gaining knowledge for the health of the entire body. Their paths may not always exude ease, but they see themselves working on something more important and satisfying than immediate gratification. Disciplined people especially use time well. They fully recognize that effective time management leads to a more disciplined life.

The danger to disciplined people lies in watching others enjoy pleasurable experiences and facing the temptation to join in. "Don't let your heart envy sinners; instead, always fear the Lord. For then you will have a future, and your hope will not be dashed" (Prov. 23:17-18). This text shows us the difference between a disciplined lifestyle choice when surrounded by those around us fulfilling their every desire and given to tasty whims. A future with hope arises as a reward of a disciplined life. When you try to do your best to live a healthy lifestyle, you have hope to live longer in good health. We know that God, at any time, can call anyone home to Heaven—whether they exude healthiness or foolishness. However, it behooves us to live our lives in such a way that we can serve our Lord.

TAMMY'S TIDBITS

It takes discipline to carry out a plan. Make a plan for tomorrow. Before you know it, you will develop the art of discipline. This art will help you in so many aspects of your life—including nutritional, physical, motivational, and spiritual fitness.

WEEK 8: DAY 5

Memory Verse: "Whoever loves discipline loves knowledge, but one who hates correction is stupid" (Prov. 12:1).

Challenge: This week, forgive yourself for making mistakes. Refocus on what you need to do, and continue on to success.

Focus: Nutritional Fitness

NATHAN'S NOTIONS

In today's devotion, we will look at those who exhibit humility. Humble people love instruction because they know there remains so much more for them to learn. Proverbs 29:23b states, "But a humble spirit will gain honor." When people stop and listen to others long enough to learn something, they show honor. When we willingly give someone else our attention and our time, we gain their trust and their honor.

I have discovered that the more I listen, the more I learn. My dad taught me some very important lessons in life. People have used the word "humble" to describe my dad's ministry. Dad told me that whenever someone called and wanted to talk to him or needed him during a crisis, he did not show up with prescribed words or a plan. He told me he said very little, and sometimes nothing at all, except for reading Scripture and praying. Dad embodied humility because he listened. The good thing about this character trait emerges as we discover that when someone learns to listen, they, in turn, learn humility. Proverbs 16:19-20 says, "Better to be lowly of spirit with the humble than to divide plunder with the proud. The one who understands a matter finds success, and the one who trusts in the LORD will be happy."

Let's apply this humble person to nutritional fitness. If someone thinks they know everything about food, they forfeit some important instruction concerning healthy eating. A humble person admits they have more to learn, will listen to good advice on eating healthily, and will incorporate what they learn into knowledge. Embrace humility. Embrace instruction. Embrace a healthier life!

TAMMY'S TIDBITS

We have a hard time saying, "I need help." First Peter 5:6-7 says, "Humble yourselves, therefore, under the mighty hand of God, so that he may exalt you at the proper time, casting all your cares on him, because he cares about you." Ask for God's help as you try to make healthy food choices.

WEEK 8: DAY 6

Memory Verse: "Whoever loves discipline loves knowledge, but one who hates correction is stupid" (Prov. 12:1).

Challenge: This week, forgive yourself for making mistakes. Refocus on what you need to do, and continue on to success.

Focus: Benefits of Friends

NATHAN'S NOTIONS

Industrious people embrace the truth that losing weight takes dedication, sweat, and tears. They do not fear the effort of counting calories, nor the sweat from exercise, nor the struggle to overcome motivational roadblocks; and they do not fear following Jesus with all their heart.

To identify industrious people according to Proverbs, we need to look at their opposite—slackers. Proverbs 21:25-26 says, "A slacker's craving will kill him because his hands refuse to work. He is filled with craving all day long, but the righteous give and don't hold back." Industrious people give everything they have to offer, holding nothing back. They do whatever it takes to accomplish their goals no matter how long it takes or how difficult the journey becomes. They see hard work as an investment in their future and do not shy away from it.

When considering the end result, we will look at Proverbs 12:27, which reads, "A lazy hunter doesn't roast his game, but to a diligent person, his wealth is precious." Industrious people find accomplishment as their reward for hard work. When we know that we have accomplished something that we could not have done by ourselves, it reminds us that friends increase efficiency. They inspire us to do more, challenge us to reach beyond our limits, and help us when we falter and fail.

Industrious people do not let failure stand in the way of success. They admit their mistake, ask and receive forgiveness for it, and carry on to a successful lifestyle change, knowing that many times, friends have helped each step of the way.

TAMMY'S TIDBITS

A good friend will support you through all your highs and lows; and as a good friend, you can do the same for others. Maybe right now, God has brought a friend to your mind that you know has a struggle. Send them a quick note of encouragement.

WEEK 8: DAY 7

Memory Verse: "Whoever loves discipline loves knowledge, but one who hates correction is stupid" (Prov. 12:1).

Challenge: This week, forgive yourself for making mistakes. Refocus on what you need to do, and continue on to success.

Challenge Carryover: As you carry this concept of forgiveness with you beyond week eight, remember that, "If we confess our sins, he is faithful and righteous to forgive us our sins and to cleanse us from all unrighteousness" (1 John 1:9). Embrace the cleansing power of forgiveness. As a child, I learned an easy way to remember what to do in case of a fire: stop, drop, and roll. Every time you make a mistake or slip just a little in your weight-loss journey, stop, drop, and pray. Stop your current actions; drop to your knees; and pray for God's forgiveness and direction to help next time you face a temptation.

Focus: Physical Fitness

NATHAN'S NOTIONS

Many benefits exist for the person who embodies discipline, humility, and industry in relation to physical fitness. Make sure to practice religiously all three of these character traits. Exhibit discipline to make time for exercise each day. Find a way. When you make it a priority, you will do it. Show humility as you ask someone for help. You may need help on learning how to perform a particular exercise or even just getting started. You may also need help in finding different ways to work the muscles of your body to maximize the potential of your exercise routines. Practice industry by diligence. Keep at it. Keep exercising. Keep turning your body into a dynamo, ready with energy to accomplish any physical task that arises.

This week, determine that you will not practice stupidity through focusing on getting your fix for food cravings, filling up with pride, or exhibiting slothfulness. Instead, choose to practice discipline, show humility, and embody industry as you serve the living Lord Jesus Christ. Make every breath you take a prayer to Him, every action you make a sacrifice to Him, and every thought you create a gift to Him. If you just imagine it, Jesus Christ can make all things possible.

TAMMY'S TIDBITS

Don't consider exercise as wasted time. Find the willpower to do some type of physical activity six days a week. Fight through the battle of the blankets, and get out of bed to exercise; you will feel so much better! Some days, you've got to dig deep, but it's there.

THIRD FOCUS: MOTIVATIONAL FITNESS

"'Everything is permissible for me,' but not everything is beneficial. 'Everything is permissible for me,' but I will not be mastered by anything" (1 Cor. 6:12).

WEEK 9: WAYS TO SUCCEED

We have discovered numerous ways to succeed in effective, permanent weight loss. They consist of setting a final goal, setting smaller goals to reach the final goal, remaining diligent, overcoming temptations, giving yourself a temporary break, learning from mistakes, not giving in to fear, and praying.

We set a final goal for successful weight loss. In your very first session, you looked at your current weight and determined a final goal. You even set a short-term goal between thirteen and twenty-six pounds for the next thirteen weeks. You have begun your journey toward successful weight loss. We encourage you to keep your final weight goal in mind as you continue this journey.

We also set smaller goals on the way. During Tammy's weight-loss journey of sixty pounds, she set three goals of twenty pounds. After she lost the first twenty, she found it easier losing another twenty. She knew she could lose that amount because she just had. When she reached the forty-pound mark, she knew she had twenty more to go. She felt as though she had just lost twenty pounds and another twenty felt like twenty too many. She then reminded herself that she had actually lost forty pounds, which sounded better and made the last twenty not so daunting.

Try dividing your total weight amount into three, four, or five smaller numbers. Even if you have a great amount of pounds to lose, breaking it into smaller amounts utilizes a great strategy. Let's say you have to lose 150 pounds. Let's break that down into five smaller amounts. That's thirty pounds. If that sounds overwhelming, then break that amount down to three goals of ten pounds or two goals of fifteen pounds. That feels more manageable. Then when you reach that small goal, set another small goal; and before you know it, you will reach that final goal.

We remained diligent with our weight-loss journey. Keep in mind, it took time to reach your current weight; it will take time to lose the weight. Normal people gain weight much easier than they lose it. No one would suffer with obesity if an easy way to lose weight existed.

Tammy found that trying to develop good habits took several days and weeks to set a good routine. And how quickly she fell back into her old unhealthy habits! Stay the course. Already you can see and feel a difference in your body. Possibly, your clothes feel a bit looser. Maybe you had to move your belt another notch in the tighter direction. You feel better because of eating healthier food. What? Could it be? You have already developed healthier habits? Good for you.

We overcame temptations. But first, you have to recognize the temptation. We have dealt with several of these in week eight. Remember, even Jesus faced temptations. He dealt with them by quoting Scripture and rebuking Satan. Stand up to temptation and say, "Not today, Satan!" Take it one day at a time.

We gave ourselves permission to take a break every once in a while. You may want to celebrate a special occasion. Go ahead and have a piece of cake—just not a HUGE piece—with all the icing. You may find that you do not like all that icing because of the overwhelming sweetness! Isn't that a horrible/wonderful way to think? You will want to watch, though, that this "break" will not turn into a Las Vegas vacation, where anything goes. When you give yourself a "break," you will also *need* to get back on a healthy course, the sooner the better.

We learned from our mistakes. The business world uses the word "challenges" for "mistakes." How will you overcome this challenge? Weight loss can become one of the most challenging things you have ever encountered.

Define your challenges. What you may see as a big challenge may not even register for another person. Refer back to weeks seven and eight for ways to overcome. If you ate too much in one meal or one day, learn to cut back on the amount of food you consume. If you ate something that made you feel bloated, then guilty, learn to remove that thing from your dietary intake! If you sat on the couch instead of going for a brisk walk, learn to overcome laziness with a motivation to reach your goal!

We did not give in to fear. "Don't be afraid" appears as the most common command in the Scriptures. Failure can make you afraid. You have told people your desire to lose weight, eat healthy, and exercise. What if they catch you cheating? What if you don't lose weight fast enough? What if you don't lose weight at all? What if . . . You fill in the blank. Rise above the fear of failure and embarrassment. Forgive yourself for making mistakes, and move on to successful weight loss.

Success can make you afraid. What if you succeed? How will your life change? We don't want to act like an annoying person who says things like, "That icing is too sweet!" "I can't eat another bite!" "I can't possibly go get ice cream; do you know how many calories that is?" "I'm so bummed I can't go running today because it is raining!"

Determine in your heart that success will not change the kind of person God has made you. Just because you no longer indulge in sweets does not mean that you do not have a sweet spirit. Just because you exercise a little now does not mean that you do not exercise good manners around the people you love. Determine that your success will not change your temperament—only your earthly tabernacle.

We prayed. Prayer helps when you find yourself overwhelmed with temptations, fear, non-compliance with what you know to do, and wavering in your goals. If you have read the devotionals, this next verse will sound familiar to you. First Peter 5:7 says, "Casting all your cares on him, because he cares about you." Jesus cares about you! And He wants all your cares. In regards to this verse, Anne Graham Lotz says, "Nothing is too mundane for God."[31] Nothing.

Because He cares for you, your weight-loss journey does not appear mundane to God. If you care about your weight loss, He cares. If you want to lose weight to give Him honor and glory, He will honor that. Pray; ask Him for help with your eating. Pray; ask Him for help with your exercise. Pray; ask Him for help with your motivation. He will honor those prayers because He cares for you!

31 Anne Graham Lotz, "God of the Impossible on 1 Peter 5:7," Daily Light for Daily Living Radio, AnGeL Ministries, Raleigh, North Carolina.

WEEK 9: DAY 1

Memory Verse: "'Everything is permissible for me,' but not everything is beneficial. 'Everything is permissible for me,' but I will not be mastered by anything."

Challenge: This week, purge your house of unhealthy foods, and/or rearrange your kitchen so that you can easily reach healthy foods, while the unhealthy ones stay out of immediate sight.

Focus: Motivational Fitness

NATHAN'S NOTIONS

As we focus on motivational fitness in today's devotional time, we want to look at judging permissible things as it relates to its helpfulness upon ourselves. When thinking about a particular action as it relates to our journey, we can ask ourselves some very pertinent questions.

Will what I do make me less spiritual? When thinking about permission from God to do all things, we have to ponder the consequences of our actions as it relates to our spiritual journey. Another way to put this question is, "Does what I intend to do help or hinder my walk with Jesus?"

Will what I do make me less useful? Whereas the previous question centered on our inner spiritual life, this one calls into focus the outward expression of our faith. If a person overeats and does not exercise, they cannot expect to serve their Lord more than if they did things that prove themselves helpful. We need to break free from this predicament and become Christ-centered in our actions.

Motivational fitness becomes crystal clear when we consider that even though all things remain permissible to us, we should focus on and do those things that makes us more spiritual and more useful. Let's exercise restraint as we keep ourselves motivated to achieving our goals.

TAMMY'S TIDBITS

Purging our kitchens of unhealthy foods helps motivate us to live healthier lifestyles. Utilize the cabinet you go to most for your healthy choices. Put your low-calorie snack choices at eye level. Do the same with the refrigerator.

WEEK 9: DAY 2

Memory Verse: "'Everything is permissible for me,' but not everything is beneficial. 'Everything is permissible for me,' but I will not be mastered by anything."

Challenge: This week, purge your house of unhealthy foods, and/or rearrange your kitchen so that you can easily reach healthy foods, while the unhealthy ones stay out of immediate sight.

Focus: Benefits of Water

NATHAN'S NOTIONS

As we look at our memory verse, we want to consider the meaning and impact of Paul's statement, "Everything is permissible for me." Taking care of the needs of the body comes forth as a natural and proper thing to do. We all have to eat and drink to survive. Instead of depriving us the joy of eating through starvation and deprivation, the Bible clearly teaches that we can enjoy, in moderation, all the good food God has provided.

Recognize that indulging in food for the purpose of satisfying our gluttony qualifies as "not everything is beneficial." Even though the verse specifically condones sexual immorality, the implication rings true. We should avoid all indulgences, for our bodies belong to the Lord.

The benefits of water guide our focus in today's devotional time. Because Paul states "everything is permissible for me," we know that we have freedom to drink whatever liquid satisfies our thirst. Nothing remains off-limits. However, we must also consider the helpfulness of what we drink and whether it will bring us under its control. Many drinks, including diet sodas, promote addictive behaviors. There remains only one best source of hydration: pure water. According to some research, drinking sufficient amounts of water daily can aid with insulin-dependent diabetes.[32] So, even though all liquids remain permissible for you to consume, choose to drink the one that stands the test of time as the most helpful: water.

TAMMY'S TIDBITS

Purge your house of unhealthy drinks. If you feel you must have soft drinks in your house, then put them in a hard-to-reach area. If possible, keep only water available as a cold drink.

---

32 Fereydoon Batmanghelidj, M.D., *Your Body's Many Cries for Water: You're Not Sick; You're Thirsty; Don't Treat Thirst with Medications* (Falls Church: Global Health Solutions, Inc., 2008), 125-27.

WEEK 9: DAY 3

Memory Verse: "'Everything is permissible for me,' but not everything is beneficial. 'Everything is permissible for me,' but I will not be mastered by anything."

Challenge: This week, purge your house of unhealthy foods, and/or rearrange your kitchen so that you can easily reach healthy foods, while the unhealthy ones stay out of immediate sight.

Focus: Spiritual Fitness

NATHAN'S NOTIONS

As we focus on spiritual fitness today, we will consider how our actions appear to God. At times, the choices we make do not consist in either good or evil; they linger between good and great. When we opt for something good, we often settle, not wanting or working toward something better, even something great.

We must look beyond matters of right and wrong when considering things helpful and consider the best possible action that will honor our Lord Jesus. The thing that may seem totally harmless and right and good at the time may, in actuality, send us on a path of wrong decisions, ultimately making that first choice wrong—like eating addictive food.

Food addiction exists just as powerful as any other addiction. As opposed to other addictions, eating seems harmless, and one can participate in the open with no fear of public ridicule. In fact, our society rewards and encourages people to over-indulge, yet condemns for over-eating and getting fat.

We all have our food addictions. I challenge you to think of spiritual fitness next time you face your addictive food and choose to love God more than your addiction. Choose to think about how you appear before God while carrying out your actions instead of satisfying your immediate desires.

TAMMY'S TIDBITS

We all face temptations like a birthday, a wedding, the Super Bowl, or Friday! When you face temptation, tell yourself you have the willpower. Remember, Jesus faced temptation and overcame; so can you with His help! And for those times you don't feel you have the willpower, pray and ask God for help to overcome.

WEEK 9: DAY 4

Memory Verse: "'Everything is permissible for me,' but not everything is beneficial. 'Everything is permissible for me,' but I will not be mastered by anything."

Challenge: This week, purge your house of unhealthy foods, and/or rearrange your kitchen so that you can easily reach healthy foods, while the unhealthy ones stay out of immediate sight.

Challenge Check-up: Have you started the purge process yet? It may seem a daunting task at first; but once you get started on it, you will discover its ease. We love a phrase Tammy learned early in her weight-loss journey: "I look better when I waste it than when I waist it." "Wasting it" may mean giving your unhealthy food away to a food pantry, so you will not have to live with the guilt of wasting food. We have grandchildren who visit us from time to time, so we have to keep some foods in the house they enjoy (for spoiling purposes). We put them up out of the way, so we do not see them or think about them until the grandkids return.

Focus: Benefits of Effective Time Management

NATHAN'S NOTIONS

Today, we want to focus on a few of the words Paul uses in our memory verse. Paul uses two words with the same root to make a point: *exestin,* translated as "is permissible," and *exousiathesomi,* translated as "mastered by."[33] The root word *exousiazo* translates as "power." In other words, "All things remain in my power, but I will not succumb to the power of any." Each of us as individuals have the power to choose things that remain helpful for us and that will not control us.

Effective time management emerges as an individual decision, yet the fact that we all have the same amount of time to use stands as a universal truth. When we embark on a path of healthy living, time bandits will always crop up. They appear as people who try to take away our time of eating healthy and exercising. Some try to rob our time intentionally, but quite honestly, most do so innocently. In practicing effective time management, seek first to understand their motivation. Learn how to say no. When someone tries to steal your time, you can always say no to the activity. There exists a great deal of freedom in saying no!

---

33 Werner Foerster, "The NT Concept of *Exousia," Theological Dictionary of the New Testament* (Grand Rapids: Wm. B. Eerdmans Publishing Company, 1964), 2:566-575.

TAMMY'S TIDBITS

Purging your house of unhealthy food requires time management. Don't try to purge the whole house of unhealthy food in one day. Choose fifteen minutes out of a day to purge unhealthy food from your eyesight to avoid temptation.

WEEK 9: DAY 5

Memory Verse: "'Everything is permissible for me,' but not everything is beneficial. 'Everything is permissible for me,' but I will not be mastered by anything."

Challenge: This week, purge your house of unhealthy foods, and/or rearrange your kitchen so that you can easily reach healthy foods, while the unhealthy ones stay out of immediate sight.

Focus: Nutritional Fitness

NATHAN'S NOTIONS

In today's devotional time with our focus on nutritional fitness, we will consider carefully the words, "But I will not be mastered by anything." Paul's anxiety about losing control under the guise of freedom comes through loud and clear. Some proclaim moral freedom through a relationship with Jesus because we live under grace instead of living under the Law. However, the pretense of moral freedom may end in moral bondage.

We should make a point to not live enslaved to any appetite or desire, however innocent. We must not allow ourselves to suffer bondage to anything. First Timothy 4:4 says, "For everything created by God is good, and nothing is to be rejected if it is received with thanksgiving." Note the caveat that Timothy includes in considering the value of everything good: received with thanksgiving. This week, as you purge your house of unhealthy food, ask yourself, "If I eat this, can I give God thanks for it?" Before you say "that's absurd" because you know you can thank God for the decadent, delicious food, think about this: how do you feel after you eat it?

After I eat delicious, nutritious food, I feel great! I feel energized; my taste buds feel satisfied; and I know I have done something that brings God glory. However, after I eat decadent food, I feel terrible! I find it very hard to give God thanks because I know that I have yielded to temptation once again. This week, choose to not let any food control your mind, mood, or meals. This week, put an end to food getting the upper hand on you, and make a point to "not be mastered by anything."

TAMMY'S TIDBITS

By this time, hopefully, you have purged your house of unhealthy foods and replaced them with healthier choices. Buy a variety of healthy food *you* like, and simply don't buy unhealthy food.

WEEK 9: DAY 6

Memory Verse: "'Everything is permissible for me,' but not everything is beneficial. 'Everything is permissible for me,' but I will not be mastered by anything."

Challenge: This week, purge your house of unhealthy foods, and/or rearrange your kitchen so that you can easily reach healthy foods, while the unhealthy ones stay out of immediate sight.

Focus: Benefits of Friends

NATHAN'S NOTIONS

In today's devotion, we will look at the benefits of friends in a different way than we have in the past weeks. We will examine how beneficial our actions appear to our friends. Paul makes it clear that he has the freedom to do all things; but in some instances, "not everything is beneficial." We have no right to do even innocent things if it causes a disadvantage to others, especially to our friends.

Whether we admit it or not, the moment we make public our desire to lose weight, we become examples. If our actions back up our words, then our examples turn into role models. However, if our examples disappoint those watching, we may send them on an unhealthy path.

"Will it help or hinder my friends?" becomes a question we should ask ourselves when making decisions about what we do on our weight-loss journey. All of us exert influence. What may seem genuinely innocent to us may serve as a devastating blow to someone who watches our actions.

A practical application for this concept includes inviting a friend to join you at a restaurant for a healthy meal. Choose carefully from the menu, setting a good example. Order a glass of water. Enjoy the meal, slowly taking time to chew thoroughly each bite, drinking water before, during, and after your meal. This week, make a conscious choice to do only things that appear helpful and beneficial to your friends.

TAMMY'S TIDBITS

A pleasant, unforeseen benefit of a friend is that they can still, without conscious effort, benefit us by helping us to eat healthier. But for me, the true test occurs when I find myself home. Alone. Freedom. I can do anything or eat anything I want. This time spent alone highlights the importance of purging our house of unhealthy food. If it ain't there, it ain't consumed.

WEEK 9: DAY 7

Memory Verse: "'Everything is permissible for me,' but not everything is beneficial. 'Everything is permissible for me,' but I will not be mastered by anything."

Challenge: This week, purge your house of unhealthy foods, and/or rearrange your kitchen so that you can easily reach healthy foods, while the unhealthy ones stay out of immediate sight.

Challenge Carryover: Hopefully by now, you have completed the purge process. From now on, pay careful attention to the food you bring into the house. Stock your pantry, freezer, and refrigerator with all kinds of nutritious and delicious foods.

Focus: Physical Fitness

NATHAN'S NOTIONS

In our focus today on physical fitness, we will look at the importance of our bodies in relation to the Lord Jesus. Paul says that he has freedom to do anything with his body as he chooses; however, he purposely chooses obedience to Christ. We can find a variety of reasons from Paul why submitting our physical fitness to the Lord qualifies as helpful.

As Christians, our bodies exist as the property of Jesus. "'Food is for the stomach and the stomach for food,' and God will do away with both of them. However, the body is not for sexual immorality but for the Lord, and the Lord for the body" (1 Cor. 6:13). Our bodies serve as conduits of God's love to the world around us, and we should avoid anything that impedes that flow. As Christians, our bodies live as members of the body of Christ. "Don't you know that your bodies are a part of Christ's body" (1 Cor. 6:15a). He uses our physical bodies to accomplish His purposes and His ways upon the earth. As Christians, our bodies serve as temples in which Jesus can dwell, reveal Himself to others, and receive worship. When we make ourselves available to the Lord, people can actually see God's love flow from our bodies.

Since our bodies belong to the Lord, we should do everything possible to present to Him the very best of ourselves. When we operate at the maximum efficiency possible with our bodies, we can serve our Lord to the best of our ability. Celebrate each victory toward your goal of a healthy lifestyle. Confess each sin of unfitness along the way. Pray; read God's Word; help others along the way; and before too long, you will serve as a role model for others as you *Imagine Not as Much*!

TAMMY'S TIDBITS

Since you have purged the house of unhealthy food, celebrate by dancing. Dance around the house; "dance like no one is looking"; dance for the joy of the Lord. King David danced. Dancing displays a great form of physical activity. Go ahead—dance, enjoy, celebrate. Have fun!

FOURTH FOCUS: SPIRITUAL FITNESS

"He must increase, but I must decrease" (John 3:30).

WEEK 10: BEGINNING A RELATIONSHIP WITH JESUS

The third focus centered on the word "Imagine" from the title of our weight loss strategy. The fourth focus will highlight the words "Not as much." The inspiration for this fourth focus comes from the words of John the Baptist that he spoke concerning the Lord Jesus Christ, which, incidentally, has nothing to do with "decreasing" in weight or waistline. Rather, John's words articulate a clear reference to the amount of influence Jesus had in his life (i.e., his wants and desires must decrease, and the wants and desires of Jesus Christ in him must increase).

We purposely began the book with nutritional and physical fitness to provide you an opportunity for successful, quick, weight loss. We continued with motivational fitness, so you could discover the "why" of what you do to lose weight. We have saved spiritual fitness until the end. We believe that spiritual fitness will serve as a key to effective, permanent weight loss, by bringing God glory through a healthier body. Once you have a healthy spiritual life through a personal relationship with Jesus Christ, everything else falls into place. Plus, if you achieve nutritional, physical, and motivational fitness, it will benefit you only while upon this earth. However, if you reach spiritual fitness, you will experience the benefits for all eternity!

We will look at "but I must decrease" in at least two different ways: decreasing in body weight and decreasing in personal wants and desires.

Quite honestly, serving the Lord Jesus Christ has inspired us to not only decrease in body weight but also to maintain our weight. In the last focus, Nathan mentioned a few things that motivated him to change his weight and, in turn, change his life. Shortening his time of ministry because of incapacitation or early death due to the complications of obesity arose as the major thing that motivated him to change. Nathan loves serving the Lord, and it grieved him that he made an unconscious decision to bring it to an early halt. He so desperately wanted Jesus to increase in his life, but he knew he must decrease in order for that to happen.

To focus on decreasing in body weight, let's look again at a powerful scriptural promise in Ephesians 3:20-21a: "Now to Him who is able to do above and beyond all that we ask or think according to the power that works in us—to him be glory."

When overweight, we do not live out the truth of this Scripture. Because we have the absolute final decision of what goes in our mouths and what we do with our bodies, we decide whether we give God glory in what we eat, drink, and do or whether to serve our own selfish desires.

We had to admit that for years we skirted around the issue of healthy eating and healthy living because we chose not to set an example of what that means. Nathan loves lasagna, chocolate, ice cream, cake (and, even better, ice cream cake), mounds of barbecued meat, loads of mashed potatoes, and piles of fried chicken (well, anything fried)! For years, he indulged himself without thinking about the impact on his body or those around him. His belly kept getting bigger, and he jokingly said, "I built a shelf to hold my books, making them easier to read."

Then in May of 2013, while reading several books about weight loss, the Holy Spirit hit Nathan between the eyeballs. He came to realize that by habitually giving in to his love for food and eating, he stood guilty before God of the sin of gluttony.

Wow! That woke him up. Nathan immediately went to the Lord in prayer and asked for God's forgiveness for his gluttony, his lack of physical activity, and his disregard for the body God had given him to inhabit while living on this earth. He decided then and there, "but I must decrease."

He also learned that his sin of gluttony contributed to obesity in his church. Everything rises and falls on leadership. When they saw their pastor overweight behind the pulpit, they felt comfortable while sitting portly in the pews.

What happens when we take seriously the sin of gluttony? What happens when we take seriously the sin of not taking care of our temples of the Holy Spirit? We come under conviction of that sin and want to do something about it. We sincerely believe that this weight loss journey to lose a few pounds acts as a living testimony of a life completely devoted to God. *Imagine Not as Much* can truly help you to achieve spiritual fitness.

To achieve spiritual fitness by decreasing in personal wants and desires, we must have a relationship with Jesus Christ. One can do that by following the Romans Road to salvation.

First, understand that we all sin by nature and by choice.

"For all have sinned and fall short of the glory of God" (**Rom. 3:23**).

Second, you can receive eternal life as a free gift.

"For the wages of sin is death, but the gift of God is eternal life in Christ Jesus our Lord" (**Rom. 6:23**).

Third, God demonstrated His love for you in a powerful, personal way.

"But God proves his own love for us in that while we were still sinners, Christ died for us" (**Rom. 5:8**).

Fourth, you must trust and surrender to Jesus as Lord.

"If you confess with your mouth, 'Jesus is Lord,' and believe in your heart that God raised him from the dead, you will be saved. One believes with the heart, resulting in righteousness, and one confesses with the mouth, resulting in salvation" (**Rom. 10:9-10**).

It's as easy as **ABC** to trust and surrender to Jesus as Lord!

Admit to God that you sin. Acts 3:19 tells us, "Therefore repent and turn back, so that your sins may be wiped out."

Believe in Jesus as the Son of God, Who can save you from your sins. Ephesians 2:8-9 states, "For you are saved by grace through faith, and this is not from yourselves; it is God's gift—not from works, so that no one can boast."

Confess Jesus Christ as Lord through prayer. The Bible has great news for you: "For everyone who calls on the name of the Lord will be saved" (Rom. 10:13).

Does what you have read make sense to you?

Can you think of any reason why you would not choose to receive God's free gift of salvation through a relationship with Jesus Christ?

Will you, right now, pray and invite Jesus Christ into your heart? If so, just say this simple prayer: "Dear Lord, I know that I sin, and I want to change. I believe in Jesus as the Son of God. I believe that You died on the cross for my sins and that You rose and live again. Please forgive me of my sins. I turn from my selfish ways and trust in You. Dear Jesus, please come into my heart and change my life. In Your precious Son's name. Amen."

WEEK 10: DAY 1

Memory Verse: "He must increase, but I must decrease" (John 3:30).

Challenge: This week, give your body to God for Him to use as He chooses.

Focus: Spiritual Fitness

NATHAN'S NOTIONS

To understand the importance and impact about John's statement about Jesus, we must know that it came from a source of joy and not obligation. The end of John 3:29 gives us the context, "So this joy of mine is complete." John exclaimed the completeness of his joy in introducing Jesus the Messiah to the world.

One can identify some basic sources for John's joy, including a more complete recognition of the person Jesus Christ. Seeing Jesus and recognizing Him as Messiah brought forth the words, "Here is the Lamb of God, who takes away the sin of the world" (John 1:29b)! Upon hearing the voice of Jesus in His teaching, John's joy escalated into spiritual ecstasy!

Another source of John's joy springs from the success of Jesus in winning the affections of those who followed Him. John's disciples complained about the success of Jesus by saying, "Rabbi, the One you testified about, and who was with you across the Jordan, is baptizing—and everyone is going to him" (John 3:26b). John did not take offense or get defensive about the success of Jesus. Instead, he rejoiced. John could see the transformation of people by their relationship with Jesus Christ. Sometimes, we get caught up in selfish thinking about our Christian walk. Once we get over the importance of ourselves, we can focus on Jesus increasing and us decreasing.

A further source of joy flows from the fulfillment of John's mission. John proclaimed the coming Messiah. He prepared the way of the Lord. Today, choose for Christ to increase in your life. Today, choose to decrease in your life. Today, choose to exercise spiritual fitness and do so because the joy of the Lord fills your heart and flows from your lips!

TAMMY'S TIDBITS

We certainly have days when we don't feel joyful. We can have joy on those days that we feel we have failed. Delve into Scripture for inspiration. Remember, "Do not grieve, because the joy of the LORD is your strength" (Neh. 8:10b).

WEEK 10: DAY 2

Memory Verse: "He must increase, but I must decrease" (John 3:30).

Challenge: This week, give your body to God for Him to use as He chooses.

Focus: Benefits of Water

NATHAN'S NOTIONS

Our memory verse speaks clearly and simply. Jesus Christ must increase in our lives, and we must decrease. We can sometimes struggle with this simple concept.

The struggle occurs when we realize the world does not revolve around us! As children, we express selfishness naturally, and this carries into our adult lives. Selfishness breeds excitement and enthusiasm over what helps us to succeed. The decision to let go of selfishness comes from within as a conscientious choice.

Paul elaborates on this inner struggle so well when he writes, "For I do not do the good that I want to do, but I practice the evil that I do not want to do" (Rom. 7:19). Even though the struggle existed for Paul, he and the ministers of the New Testament purposely hid themselves behind the greater glory of their Lord—the same thing we must do. No matter how considerable our abilities and powers, they only engage serviceability as they contribute to the glory of Christ.

A matter of trust identifies another cause for the struggle to let Jesus increase and us to decrease. Do we trust that Jesus knows the best for us? Do we trust that Jesus can take the lead in our lives on His own without any help from us? When we answer honestly those questions in our hearts, the struggle ceases; and we will yield to Jesus.

Today's devotional centers on the benefits of water. Drinking the appropriate amount of water carries with it many health benefits. When we trust that water will benefit us greatly, we will drink it regularly. In the same way, when we trust that Jesus can handle our lives better than we can, we will yield to Him joyfully and completely. After all, as servants of the most High King, we simply act as forerunners, preparing others to experience a relationship with Jesus.

TAMMY'S TIDBITS

One health benefit of water includes treatment of frequent heartburn.[34] The next time you experience heartburn, try drinking eight ounces of water.

---

34 Ibid, 27.

WEEK 10: DAY 3

Memory Verse: "He must increase, but I must decrease" (John 3:30).

Challenge: This week, give your body to God for Him to use as He chooses.

Focus: Nutritional Fitness

NATHAN'S NOTIONS

As we think about our memory verse this week, let's consider the broader consistency of John's testimony. His testimony was identified by what his role did not consist of, what his role included, and the evidence of his persistence in proclaiming his role. John purposely pointed people to Jesus, knowing he himself did not fulfill the role of Messiah.

John knew his role as the forerunner for the Messiah. Everything we do should point people to Jesus instead of ourselves. John did so naturally and effortlessly; so must we. John practiced consistency in his life in regards to Jesus' influence increasing and his influence decreasing.

Our focus today centers on nutritional fitness. When we eat, we can embody the same characteristics of John. We can know that our role upon this earth as born-again Christians does not consist of simply gorging ourselves to satisfy our own personal gluttony.

We can know our role as an example to a watching world, so that everything we do should point people to Jesus. When we overeat, the spotlight focuses on us instead of Jesus.

We can consistently eat responsibly, so our bodies will give glory to God. As we learned previously, our bodies need only ten times our weight in calories to sustain normal daily activities. When we eat above that amount, the excess turns into waste and/or fat. If you will eat ten times your target weight in calories each day, you will lose weight. Decide you will exercise responsible nutritional fitness with each meal and snack you eat every day. Today, choose to purposely decrease in calorie intake so the light of Jesus can increase in your life!

TAMMY'S TIDBITS

Make sure to measure your food. How can you do that consistently? Start each day by planning what you will eat for the day. Then record your meals and snacks. Did they match for the day? Good for you! If they did not, watch for opportunities and challenges. Before you know it, consistency will become a normal part of your life, and your life will point others to Jesus.

WEEK 10: DAY 4

Memory Verse: "He must increase, but I must decrease" (John 3:30).

Challenge: This week, give your body to God for Him to use as He chooses.

Challenge Check-up: Have you yielded your body to God? This week, concentrate on seeing your body as an instrument in the hand of God to be used for His glory. You will gain the joy of knowing that God works in you and through you, touching lives around you!

Focus: Benefits of Effective Time Management

NATHAN'S NOTIONS

Let's consider what it means for Jesus to increase in our lives and for us to decrease. We begin with an understanding that when we decrease, we do not minimize ourselves; but we make our scope of influence narrower so the influence of Jesus can grow wider. Since Jesus claims Himself as King, our role becomes that of a servant. If we think that role has no value, we should remember that Jesus notices every servant of His. Today, as a servant of the Most High King, give all you have to Him, including your time.

We ask that you consider continuing the *Imagine Not as Much* journey as an Imaginator. An Imaginator is one who has read the book and/or participated in a group and, because of his/her experience, wants to share this knowledge with others. You might object, and we understand the hesitancy. However, one benefit consists of knowing that as someone looks to you as an example and depends upon you for inspiration, it will help you tremendously to stay focused. An additional benefit comes when you see someone else's life begin to transform because of your influence.

Today's focus centers on benefits of effective time management. Accepting the challenge of serving as an Imaginator will take time. Investing in the life of someone else to help them grow in their relationship with Jesus, along with seeing their overall attitude improve as they lose weight, qualifies as one of the most significant uses of your time.

When you experience grace bestowed upon someone brokenhearted over weight issues, your desire will deepen for Jesus to increase and for you to decrease for the glory of God!

TAMMY'S TIDBITS

I keep thinking of the widow with her two tiny coins and how she gave out of her poverty all she had to God. In a way, we all have a lack of time—a poverty of time, if you will. I wonder if we gave our poverty of time to serve Him, would we miss it? Go ahead and try today to spend your free time serving the Lord.

WEEK 10: DAY 5

Memory Verse: "He must increase, but I must decrease" (John 3:30).

Challenge: This week, give your body to God for Him to use as He chooses.

Focus: Physical Fitness

NATHAN'S NOTIONS

Today's devotional will focus on the word "must" and how that word applies to physical fitness. The word "must" has different connotations, depending upon the context.

One connotation occurs when someone says the word to us, either as a command or an ultimatum. Another connotation occurs when we ourselves use the word "must." We understand the urgency and importance of the task at hand and attach a "must" to motivate ourselves to complete it. You may have enrolled in class because you had a "must" moment about your unhealthy weight. Someone else's "must" cannot motivate you to continue. Permanent weight loss does not come easy. It takes hard work, dedication, and time. Effective weight loss can happen only if the "must" comes from within you.

The most effective way to lose weight and keep it off is through physical fitness. When we engage in physical fitness, we turn our bodies into calorie-burning machines. Every pound of fat that turns to muscle burns more calories, so even the simple things we do help us lose weight.

If you do not currently engage in physical fitness, listen to your "must." If your "must" to lose weight becomes strong in your spirit, you will get off the couch and get moving. When your "must" reaches a critical point in your life, you will exercise. As you participate in physical fitness, your body will get stronger; your breathing will get better; and your overall self-confidence will improve.

TAMMY'S TIDBITS

I suggest that in addition to some sort of cardio, add some weight-lifting to your activity. This could consist of something as simple as lifting small weights (or even cans) for a few minutes every day.

WEEK 10: DAY 6

Memory Verse: "He must increase, but I must decrease" (John 3:30).

Challenge: This week, give your body to God for Him to use as He chooses.

Focus: Benefits of Friends

NATHAN'S NOTIONS

Today's devotion will look at the reasons behind John's statement about Jesus, beginning with the relationship of Jesus to other believers. Jesus takes on the identity of the Groom, and the Church the identity of the Bride. His claim stands because no other valid Groom exists. Jesus alone came from eternity, inhabited human flesh, lived a perfect life, died on the cross, and rose again. Only Jesus can save people from their sins. His claim also stands because Jesus' coming to the earth expresses God's love for all humanity. His sacred life provided the perfect sacrifice of the Lamb of God Who takes away the sin of the world.

Another reason for John's statement springs from his relationship with Jesus as his friend. John could have accepted the attention of the crowd, but he knew that would not make him the friend of Jesus, but His foe.

We may call Jesus Teacher, Rabbi, or Son of God. However, if we cannot call Him our Friend, then we have not entered into a relationship with Him as Savior. Today's devotion focuses on the benefits of friends. In order for your journey to succeed, you need friends who also know Jesus as Friend to help you along the way. Get involved in a local church that can help you lose weight. A local church epitomizes a group of friends who love you and want to help you.

You can count on your friends in class to help you achieve your weight loss goal. You can expect them to pray with you, to discuss what works in their lives for effective weight loss with you, to laugh with you about the funny things that happen along your journey, and to cry with you during difficult times.

TAMMY'S TIDBITS

Friends enhance any journey worth having, including this one for weight loss. Invite a friend to church. You may feel reluctant going to church; however, a friend can make it easier and more enjoyable.

WEEK 10: DAY 7

Memory Verse: "He must increase, but I must decrease" (John 3:30).

Challenge: This week, give your body to God for Him to use as He chooses.

Challenge Carryover: The carryover is the same as the challenge. Each day, each week, give your body to God for Him to use as He chooses. I guarantee you will not regret it!

Focus: Motivational Fitness

NATHAN'S NOTIONS

Today's devotion will look at John's private thoughts before he spoke the words in our memory verse. When the disciples tattled on the events surrounding Jesus baptizing, "John responded, 'No one can receive anything unless it has been given to him from heaven'" (John 3:27). John knew his role and that of the Messiah were gifts from a merciful God. He decided to look at things from God's perspective. John warded off jealousy and rivalry. He realized that everything he had came from God. Because of Divine harmony, there existed no need for him to express jealously, pride, or dejection in comparing his work with that of Jesus. He realized both he and Jesus operated exactly the way the Heavenly Father intended: he as the herald, and Jesus as the Messiah.

We, too, can experience the freedom John experienced. We can remember that God has a plan and purpose for every person. We can rise above jealousy and rivalry. While on this journey, someone will lose weight faster, and someone will lose weight slower. When either of these scenarios occur, our response might include jealousy, rivalry, pride, or hurt feelings. When we keep in mind our focus, we can stay motivated to reach our goal. Without that focus, we can get easily derailed, discouraged, and eventually quit the journey. However, we can stay on track.

By releasing our tendency to feel jealous over someone else's success and pride when they do better, we set ourselves free to celebrate and comfort others. When we see things as God sees them, we see that everything works in harmony to accomplish His plan. This week, stay motivated; stay strong; and stay connected to Jesus. Completely yield to Him, and you will experience a life-long journey of healthy living.

TAMMY'S TIDBITS

How does one stay motivated when others on the same journey achieve more success? We can do a couple of things: either throw ourselves a pity party or pick ourselves up, dust ourselves off, and keep on keepin' on! Trust in yourself. Rejoice for others; and know that if you remain consistent, you will succeed.

FOURTH FOCUS: SPIRITUAL FITNESS

"The one who sent me is with me. He has not left me alone, because I always do what pleases him"

(John 8:29).

WEEK 11: DEVELOPING A LIFE-LONG RELATIONSHIP WITH JESUS

Just as obesity indicates an unhealthy relationship with food, spiritual unfitness indicates an unhealthy relationship with God. Spiritual fitness involves more than a one-time decision made some time ago. Spiritual fitness cultivates a life-long relationship with Jesus Christ. You can enhance that life-long relationship by doing a number of simple yet powerful things: accepting Jesus Christ as Savior, finding a good church home, reading the Bible every day, studying the Bible every week, praying every day, and sharing with someone God's work in your life.

Accept God's free gift of salvation through confessing Jesus Christ as Lord through prayer. Without this first vital step you cannot continue to develop a relationship with Jesus. You must know Him as Savior to eventually make Him Lord over all your life.

Perhaps you are reading the *Imagine Not as Much* book but have not participated in a group—either because you have not found one or because you felt uncomfortable joining one with people you did not know. You have probably experienced some success in your weight loss. Nathan lost thirty pounds all by himself. So why do we encourage you to find or start an Imagine Not as Much group? Because of the benefits you will receive. We will unpack these benefits later as they relate to a good church home.

Find a good church home. If you already belong to a good church family, begin inviting people to church. Many people would start attending if only asked. If they say no, it's not the end of the world. Keep at it—someone may surprise you and say yes!

Attending church will help you in your spiritual fitness in many of the same ways as does attending your Imagine Not as Much group. These include support, encouragement, accountability, fellowship, learning something new, and finding a purpose.

Hopefully you have found support with your leaders and fellow class members. The same rings true at a good church. You will find many pastors and other church leaders who have a true heart for people and would love to help others through the struggles of every-day life. Sometimes, you just need a listening ear, and you can find that in a good church that has compassionate, caring people.

Without a shadow of a doubt, you have faced discouragement about some portion of your weight loss journey. Perhaps the weight didn't come off one week like you expected or hoped, or perhaps temptation got the best of you and proper nutrition did not make your top ten priority list. Perhaps you just felt unmotivated to exercise. But something made you go to class, and you found encouragement either from the leader or a fellow Imaginator. You can and will find this same kind of encouragement with a good church family. When you feel discouraged, tempted, non-motivated, or like giving up, a church leader or fellow member may have just the right word or actions that will encourage you beyond measure.

Accountability offered a strong reason to keep coming back to class. You knew you needed a little extra push after an extra hard week. Attending church can provide the same accountability. A good church will encourage you to walk the straight and narrow path by hearing God's Word and making practical applications to everyday life.

Perhaps you made friends with people that you would have never met aside from the Imagine Not as Much group. Who knew that someone else struggled the same way you do and shared similar thoughts and temptations? Not so surprisingly, you can find friends in a good church home, where you can expect a sweet, sweet fellowship.

We hope that by now in your reading of *Imagine Not as Much*, you have learned something new. Accordingly, attending Sunday School and worship offers opportunities every Sunday to learn something new. God speaks in new and refreshing ways on a weekly basis. He does this as you attend Sunday school class, studying His Word in a small group atmosphere. He continues to speak through the singing and preaching of the Word in the worship hour. Sunday morning presents a great time for experiencing a living, loving God.

Belonging to a church will also give us a purpose. Just as the Imagine Not as Much class gives you something to look forward to, you can eagerly anticipate Sunday mornings. You have unique gifts that may help the church or others in astounding ways. The thought never crossed our minds that losing weight would lead to a ministry opportunity. Nothing exists outside the realms of possibility with God.

Read the Bible every day. Bookstores carry several versions of the Bible. Find one that you like that's easy to read. We use the Christian Standard Bible version in *Imagine Not as Much*, but many others exist. Buy tabs that have the books of the Bible, and put them in your Bible, making them easy to find. Tammy uses tabs even today. Underline passages that speak to you. Yes, the Bible is holy; but when you underline a passage, it can offer encouragement at a later date.

Find a time for reading the Bible that works best for you, utilizing effective time management. The *Imagine Not as Much* devotions address time management one day a week. Find a time to do your devotion. Tammy has found that after her and Nathan's morning walk and her shower, that breakfast and the Bible go well together. Even though as a pastor Nathan reads the Bible daily to prepare for his sermons and Bible studies, he also sets aside time in the mornings for his own personal time with the Lord.

Study the Bible every week. The difference between reading and studying the Bible involves taking notes on what impacts you and making a commitment to put into practice what you learn. Sunday school serves as a great place to study the Bible with a group of people and make new friends. You can also study the Bible at home. You can study books of the Bible, people of the Bible, or doctrines found in the Bible, to name just a few areas of study.

Study takes time and energy. Paul encourages us to make time and expend energy when he writes in 2 Timothy 2:15, "Be diligent to present yourself to God as one approved, a worker who doesn't need to be ashamed, correctly teaching the word of truth." One way to present yourself as approved to God includes memorizing Scripture. Our devotion for this week includes tips on how to memorize. Memorizing the Bible reference holds just as much importance as the Bible verse, so you can find it when someone asks you, "Where does it say that in the Bible?"

Pray every day. Spend alone time with God, talking with Him and listening to what He says to you through the Holy Spirit. Tammy has found her drive to work in the mornings a great time to have a talk with the Lord. Nathan relishes his alone time in the office every morning as time to meet the Lord in prayer.

Share with someone else what God has done in your life. You can use your experience in your weight loss journey as a bridge to do just that. We will talk about this more in our next session.

WEEK 11: DAY 1

Memory Verse: "The one who sent me is with me. He has not left me alone, because I always do what pleases him" (John 8:29).

Challenge: This week, make a point to memorize Scripture.

Focus: Spiritual Fitness

NATHAN'S NOTIONS

In today's devotional time, we will consider the statement of Jesus, "I always do what pleases him." This statement represents the dedication and devotion of Jesus to the will of God the Father as evidenced in His incarnation. Jesus began His journey of pleasing the Father before He came to Earth and continued to do so even as a child. He pleased the Father as an obscure carpenter's Son: "The boy grew up and became strong, filled with wisdom, and God's grace was on him" (Luke 2:40). Jesus continued to please the Father throughout His entire life, not because He had to, but because it brought Him great delight.

Jesus pleased the Father by fulfilling the ceremonial law, by obedience to the moral law, and by His prayers. He pleased the Father in His crucifixion, resurrection, and ascension. He will please the Father in His coming again. Jesus had a keen sense of the presence of God the Father because everywhere, at all times, He did and said what pleased the Father.

As we focus on spiritual fitness today, we, too, can have a keen awareness of the presence of God in our lives by purposely trying to please the Father in all that we do, including what we eat and drink. God cares about us. When we focus on pleasing Him, we sense His presence and experience His peace.

Know that you do not have to walk your weight loss journey alone. You can have the sense and awareness that God has not left you alone if you listen to His voice and obey His promptings. Today, choose obedience, and experience His presence with every step of your weight-loss journey.

TAMMY'S TIDBITS

Memorizing Scripture serves as one way to please God. Try these few tips that might help. First, break down the verse into smaller portions. Our memory verse easily breaks down into three different parts: 1) "The one who sent me is with me," 2) "He has not left me alone," and 3) "Because I always do what pleases him." Second, highlight key words in each section. Highlight "One who sent," "not left me," and "always pleases." Third, keep the verse where you can see it daily. More tips to come!

WEEK 11: DAY 2

Memory Verse: "The one who sent me is with me. He has not left me alone, because I always do what pleases him" (John 8:29).

Challenge: This week, make a point to memorize Scripture.

Focus: Benefits of Water

NATHAN'S NOTIONS

Yesterday's devotion looked at the general principle of doing what pleases the Father. Today, we will consider some practical applications of the principle. The word in our memory verse—"always"—will guide our thoughts today.

We can practice obedience to God "always" by paying attention to the relationships around us, our obligations, and opportunities that present a choice. We can make every attempt to show God's love in our relationships around us. It seems that we have the ability to show the love of Christ to everyone else except for those closest to us, especially those with whom we do life.

We can also please God in practical ways as we fulfill our obligations joyfully and to the best of our abilities. There should never exist a halfhearted effort on our part in anything we do, but only the best effort. That includes drinking water. As we focus on the benefits of water today, we can remember that some research reveals that gastritis can be treated with drinking sufficient amounts of water each day.[35]

When we strive to please the Father "always," we try to make choices pleasing to Him as opportunities present themselves. We all make choices. Some choices seem easy, while others seem difficult. Every choice has a consequence. Opportunities for choices frequently occur in the unexpected, when things happen that we did not think about. We can either please the Father or displease the Father with the choices that we make.

TAMMY'S TIDBITS

I almost "always" drink water, with exception to my coffee first thing in the morning. I can tell a huge difference in the way I feel when I do not drink enough water. I wish I "always" memorized the weekly Scripture verse. I feel unprepared to talk with people about spiritual things when I have not memorized Scripture. Repetition represents a fourth tip for memorizing Scripture. Repeat the key phrases several times.

---

35 Ibid, 27.

WEEK 11: DAY 3

Memory Verse: "The one who sent me is with me. He has not left me alone, because I always do what pleases him" (John 8:29).

Challenge: This week, make a point to memorize Scripture.

Focus: Nutritional Fitness

NATHAN'S NOTIONS

Today's devotion will look at multifarious things which displease the Father, so we can make an effort to avoid them: pride, slothfulness, carelessness, anger, unbelief, and murmuring.

Pride displeases the Father, whether we flaunt our talent, self-righteousness, wealth, or rank. Pride pulls our focus away from God and places it upon ourselves, making us more important than God.

Slothfulness or slackness cheats others from receiving the very best of our efforts. We discredit God when we do not put forth our best effort at serving Him.

Carelessness resembles slothfulness in that it conveys an attitude of, "I just don't care." When we exhibit carelessness, we displease God because we take lightly what has cost God the Father greatly: His Son, Jesus.

There remain times and events for righteous anger; but on the whole, anger displeases God. When anger boils in our spirit, it often bubbles over in words and ways that dishonor His name. Unbelief displeases the Father when we do not believe that God loves us, that God knows best, or that we cannot do what God calls us to do.

Unbelief happens when people don't attempt a healthy lifestyle through nutritional fitness. When told the amount of calories one needs to lose weight, two extreme forms of unbelief surface. One, they do not believe they can lose weight by eating that many calories. Or two, they believe they cannot exist on that few of calories. Do not let unbelief keep you from achieving success in nutritional fitness.

The last thing entails murmuring, complaining under your breath about something with which you disagree. It avoids truth and, thus, displeases God greatly.

If you have trouble sensing God's presence with you each day, check to see if any of these things influence your life. If they do, recognize it; confess it; turn away from it; keep it out of your life; and give your heart to pleasing the Father.

TAMMY'S TIDBITS

All the things that Nathan mentioned dissuade us from memorizing Scripture. But it pleases God greatly when we do. Try repeating this week's memory verse one phrase at a time.

WEEK 11: DAY 4

Memory Verse: "The one who sent me is with me. He has not left me alone, because I always do what pleases him" (John 8:29).

Challenge: This week, make a point to memorize Scripture.

Challenge Check-up: Have you begun memorizing Scripture this week? If not, make time today to focus on the memory verse. John 8:29 constitutes a short verse with a powerful message. You have had eleven memory verses so far, and we pray you will have success as you hide each one of them in your heart!

Focus: Benefits of Effective Time Management

NATHAN'S NOTIONS

In today's devotional, we will look at the statement, "The one who sent me is with me." Jesus always felt the presence of the Father. We can also experience a real knowledge of God's presence.

We enjoy God's presence by a unity of essence. When we accept Jesus into our hearts as Lord, we come to know God in intimate ways because God dwells in our lives. Our essence becomes changed by His essence.

We are aware of God's presence by a communion of spirit. When we work on our relationship with God, we begin to want to know Him in an intimate way and to let His Spirit lead us.

We experience God's presence in a consciousness of favor. When we trust and obey God, we can sense a special measure of His favor upon us. When we effectively manage our time enjoying the favor of God, it gives us more free time to do things that please Him, not because we have to, but because we want to.

We understand God's presence by His present help. We know that God's help exists with just praying. When we walk with the Lord, we know His help stands ready.

We participate with God's presence through His eternal plans. We see eternity differently than we used to and differently than those who do not know the Lord. We want to make it our mission to tell others about how they can experience peace with God in Heaven.

Memorizing Scripture helps us to understand our unity of essence with the Father, experience the communion of His Spirit, stay conscious of His favor, know the immediacy of His help, and focus on eternal things. Make a point to memorize Scripture and make Jesus' scriptural promise yours.

TAMMY'S TIDBITS

Make time every day to write down the memory verse ten times to aid in your memorization.

WEEK 11: DAY 5

Memory Verse: "The one who sent me is with me. He has not left me alone, because I always do what pleases him" (John 8:29).

Challenge: This week, make a point to memorize Scripture.

Focus: Physical Fitness

NATHAN'S NOTIONS

Physical fitness guides our focus today. When we think of using our bodies for God's glory, we can see how the way we conduct ourselves translates into holiness. Holiness shows the depth of our devotion and commitment to the one true God. We live our lives for His glory. In other words, we "play for an audience of one."

Jamey Carroll made his Big League debut in 2002. A native of Evansville, Indiana, he found success through his aggressive, crowd-pleasing style as an infielder.[36] While playing for the Washington Nationals, he commented on his style of play by saying, "If I can be a light in this field that somebody in the stands can see Christ through me, that's truly the reason I go out and I play for Him."[37] Jamey exemplified holiness in playing for an audience of one. We can, too, as we pursue a healthy lifestyle through physical fitness. We can make choices daily that reflect God's glory. Holiness exists as a gift from God to those who truly want to live for Him.

As we embrace holiness, we can know the truth of the words of Jesus in our memory verse. The holiness we express does not really come from us but from God, just like sunbeams emanate from the sun. God shines; we reflect. We experience and share the warmth of His love because of His work flowing in and through us. Today, choose to make your physical activities conduits of the truth of God's love while you conduct yourself in obedient holiness!

TAMMY'S TIDBITS

Learning the "address" of a Scripture verse offers the opportunity to open the Bible and share the verse with someone. We can also view the surrounding verses and learn new concepts. Referencing the book, chapter, and verse remains a very important part of any memory verse. Right now, say the reference "address" for this week's memory verse without looking.

---

36 Wikipedia, "Jamey Carroll, Wikipedia.com, en.wikipedia.org/wiki/Jamey_Carroll, (accessed August 1, 2015).
37 CBN, "Playing for an Audience of One," CBN.com, http://www1.cbn.com/sports/jamey-carroll%3A-playing-for-an-audience-of-one (accessed August 1, 2015).

WEEK 11: DAY 6

Memory Verse: "The one who sent me is with me. He has not left me alone, because I always do what pleases him" (John 8:29).

Challenge: This week, make a point to memorize Scripture.

Focus: Benefits of Friends

NATHAN'S NOTIONS

As we think about the benefits of friends in our devotional time today, let's look at 1 Corinthians 12:18, which reads, "But as it is, God has arranged each one of the parts in the body just as he wanted." The body of which 1 Corinthians alludes describes the Church. This verse tells us something significant about all the unique types of people brought together as a Church. God placed them in the Body, the Church, just as He wanted so they could receive help along their spiritual journey and so they could help others along in their spiritual journeys.

God has drawn you to join Imagine Not as Much through your church for the same reasons. There will come a time that you will need help to lose and/or maintain a healthy weight. On difficult weeks, God has placed you among a group that understands your struggles and stands ready to help you along the way. At other times, you will have the opportunity to share how you got around and/or over a struggle.

God—Who knows you and loves you—has brought you into this group with a purpose. He has surrounded you with friends who have the same goal in mind. Your friends will help you stay on track, and you will help others do the same. God has sent you here, and He has not left you alone. He uses people around you to show you His love and care for you.

TAMMY'S TIDBITS

Make a game out of memorizing the verse by writing each word on a separate piece of paper. Then shuffle and give them to your friend to place on a table in random order. Next, have your friend check your accuracy as you place the words in the correct order.

WEEK 11: DAY 7

Memory Verse: "The one who sent me is with me. He has not left me alone, because I always do what pleases him" (John 8:29).

Challenge: This week, make a point to memorize Scripture.

Challenge Carryover: Keep trying to memorize Scripture. God's Word will guide you and direct you each day.

Focus: Motivational Fitness

NATHAN'S NOTIONS

Today, for our focus on motivational fitness, we will consider a handful of simple things Jesus did which we can also do to embody the "do" of our memory verse. One thing that Jesus did was pray. First Thessalonians 5:17 tells us to "pray constantly." We can take on the spirit of prayer throughout our entire day and spend time in concentrated prayer when alone.

Another thing that Jesus did was love the Father and mankind. He obeyed the Father out of His love for Him and His love for the world. We love the Father as we obey Him and present our bodies as living sacrifices to Him, and we love mankind as we share with them the Good News of salvation through Jesus.

Jesus also remained separate from sinners, yet engaged them in compassion. He lived a perfect, sinless life while here upon the earth yet took time to show and share the love of the Father to sinners. To follow His example, we must not conform to this world, but yet must stay engaged in the world, so sinners can come to a saving knowledge of Jesus.

Our motivational fitness will grow strong as we pray, as we love the Father and mankind, and as we stay separate yet engaged with sinners. Pray specifically for God to use you to show His love to others around you. Pray for a deeper relationship with Him and a broader scope of compassion for those who do not yet know Him. And pray that as people witness your weight loss, they will give God glory for His work in your life!

TAMMY'S TIDBITS

As we come to the close of this week's devotion and memorizing this week's verse, we can stand encouraged with the hard work. For some, memorizing appears easy, while for others it creates a struggle. What else does that sound like? Did you struggle this week with nutritional and physical fitness, or did everything fall easily into place? Take the tools of memorizing Scripture and see how it relates to a healthier lifestyle. We set our goal (ideal weight, memory verse); we make a plan (plan each meal, divide into phrases); and we work hard to achieve results.

FOURTH FOCUS: SPIRITUAL FITNESS

"But in your hearts regard Christ the Lord as holy, ready at any time to give a defense to anyone who asks you for a reason for the hope that is in you" (1 Peter 3:15).

WEEK 12: USING IMAGINE NOT AS MUCH TO SHARE YOUR RELATIONSHIP WITH JESUS

To focus on decreasing in personal wants and desires, let's look at how you can use *Imagine Not as Much* to reach your friends, family, and neighbors with the Gospel of Jesus Christ. Simply put, when they ask how you have lost weight, you have an answer for them. You can tell them you took a thirteen-week class or read the book entitled *Imagine Not as Much* that helped you focus on four areas of fitness.

Just how does one do that? We're so glad you asked! We have come up with an acronym for IMAGINE to help you discuss your weight loss with others.

Imagine

Made

Achieve

Group

Invite

Needed

Empowered

You can say, "***Imagine*** *Not as Much* was the title of a book I read that **Made** me realize that I could **Achieve** success in weight loss. It encourages a **Group** setting to learn about four different types of fitness and give support to each other. I **Invite** you to join me in a class. I found the help I **Needed** to lose weight, and *Imagine Not as Much* has **Empowered** me to live a healthy lifestyle and maintain my weight loss for the rest of my life."

If someone asks you any type of spiritual question, you can lead the conversation to a point where you can share your story. You have a unique story and a shared story.

Your unique story emerges from the truth that God made only one of you, and He loves you just the way He made you. You have different physical attributes than anyone on the face of planet Earth and a personality all your own.

Your shared story merges with everyone else's who has accepted God's invitation to join His family through a personal relationship with Jesus Christ. Through inviting Jesus into your heart as Savior, you gain a multitude of brothers and sisters in Christ, all sharing the same story of salvation in Jesus!

We want you to feel comfortable sharing your salvation story. You can effectively tell someone your story in these simple steps: your life before Jesus, how you accepted Jesus as Savior, and your life since you accepted Jesus.

Your life before Jesus briefly details a little about your thoughts, actions, and feelings before you accepted Jesus. You do not have to share graphic details in this part of your story, nor make it lengthy. Doing either will only glorify Satan. Just give a brief summary.

How you accepted Jesus as Savior describes the event of your salvation experience. You may not remember the exact day; but if you have passed from darkness to light, from death to life, you will remember the event. Tell the circumstances surrounding your prayer to invite Jesus into your heart: the who, what, where, when, and why.

Whereas the previous steps recount past events, so the descriptions do not change; telling the next step about your life since you accepted Jesus has the potential to change daily. Keep this step of telling your story current by sharing the blessings you encounter because of your personal relationship with Jesus. This step of telling your story lends itself nicely to talking about your Imagine Not as Much weight loss journey. You can explain to someone that you view this journey not just as a way to lose a few pounds, but also as a way to honor God with your body.

Pray for opportunities to let someone know about your weight loss journey and the chance to tell your story about a personal relationship with Jesus Christ.

Stay aware that people you know watch you. They watch what you say, what you do, where you go, and what you eat. Make every effort to make sure that what they see when they watch you glorifies God and gives you an opening to tell your story.

Invite those who ask you how you lost weight to join you in an Imagine Not as Much class. Intentionally use your Imagine Not as Much experience as a way to glorify God with your body, seeing it as an opportunity to pursue spiritual fitness. If they show interest in taking the class, offer to take it with them, helping as an Imaginator until they reach their goal.

If you belong to a current class of Imagine Not as Much, next week you will have your celebration meal. Everyone will be asked to bring a healthy dish and its recipe to share with the class. Think of someone you could invite.

Record their name: _____

Also consider assisting as an Imaginator for someone who may join the class from the community. View Imagine Not as Much as a great way to find a new friend, give them an opportunity to experience new life in Jesus Christ, and help disciple them to grow deeper in their relationship with the Lord.

WEEK 12: DAY 1

Memory Verse: "But in your hearts regard Christ the Lord as holy, ready at any time to give a defense to anyone who asks you for a reason for the hope that is in you" (1 Peter 3:15).

Challenge: This week, share your story with someone who has not heard it.

Focus: Spiritual Fitness

NATHAN'S NOTIONS

In today's focus during our devotional time, let's look at what this means: "But in your hearts regard Christ the Lord as holy." "Regard" in our memory verse comes from the Greek word *hagiasate*, which means to sanctify or set apart for holiness.[38] In this text, Peter draws from the words of the prophet Isaiah as recorded in chapter eight verse thirteen: "You are to regard only the Lord of Armies as holy. Only he should be feared; only he should be held in awe."

Before we explore the meaning of this word, we must first look at what it does *not* mean. God stands most holy in and of Himself, and thus we cannot make Him holy in our lives. God embodies holiness in its fullest expression by simply existing.

The phrase "in your hearts regard Christ the Lord as holy" means that we set Him apart as holy in our hearts. As Christians, this act of setting apart the Messiah should come easily and often. When we set apart the Messiah as Lord, each moment of the day becomes an opportunity to experience God. The ordinary becomes extraordinary as we see God in the details of life. We see the people in our sphere of influence become possible recipients of the love of God flowing through us. We see the quiet times in our day as invitations to converse with God. We can read and meditate upon His Word, reflecting on how He has used us in His service. We can also prepare ourselves for service again.

View your actions as sacred touches of God upon others. Consider your words as sacred utterances of God to inspire and help others. Give even the smallest detail of your life to the sacredness of God's presence!

TAMMY'S TIDBITS

This week, pray about sharing your story. Pray that God will give you the words to say and the courage to speak. Pray for the person whom God places in your path to share your story.

---

38 Otto Procksch, "*Hagios* in the N.T." *Theological Dictionary of the New Testament* (Grand Rapids: Wm. B. Eerdmans Publishing Company, 1964), 1:100-115.

WEEK 12: DAY 2

Memory Verse: "But in your hearts regard Christ the Lord as holy, ready at any time to give a defense to anyone who asks you for a reason for the hope that is in you" (1 Peter 3:15).

Challenge: This week, share your story with someone who has not heard it.

Focus: Benefits of Water

NATHAN'S NOTIONS

Today's devotion will look at the phrase from our memory verse, "the hope that is in you," as it pertains to future things. Hope of eternal life lives in the hearts of Christians. We have confident hope that this side of eternity—mortality—will not continue forever. We have confident hope that because we repented of our sins, believed in Jesus as the Son of God, and called upon Him as Lord through prayer that we have a home waiting for us in Heaven. If you do not have this hope, make yourself right with God today. Confess and repent of your sin, believe in Jesus, and invite Him into your heart through prayer. Hope is a powerful feeling that empowers all we say and all we do each day until we see Jesus.

As we focus on the benefits of water today, we can incorporate this idea of a hope of future things. One of the benefits we gain from drinking water comes in how it affects our bodies in the long-term or, if you will, the future. For instance, some research has shown that sufficient water aids with arthritis and rheumatoid arthritis.[39]

TAMMY'S TIDBITS

Today, as we talk about sharing our story with others and the benefits of water, I can't help but think of Jesus, Who shared His story with the woman at the well. He said in John 4:14, "But whoever drinks from the water that I will give him will never get thirsty again. In fact, the water I will give him will become a well of water springing up in him for eternal life." Just as Jesus shared with the woman as she gathered water for her daily needs, so we can share our stories about Jesus' work in our lives by drinking water every day and losing weight.

---

39 Reynolds, 135.

WEEK 12: DAY 3

Memory Verse: "But in your hearts regard Christ the Lord as holy, ready at any time to give a defense to anyone who asks you for a reason for the hope that is in you" (1 Peter 3:15).

Challenge: This week, share your story with someone who has not heard it.

Focus: Nutritional Fitness

NATHAN'S NOTIONS

In today's devotion time, we will consider again the words from our memory verse, "the hope that is in you." Hope evokes the rich and excellent blessings that God gives to His believers.

When I began my journey of permanent weight loss in May 2013, something changed inside of me that I had not experienced in my previous attempts to lose weight. I saw my weight loss as a way to honor God and as a way to please Him.

As we focus on nutritional fitness today, we can have hope that what we eat makes a big difference in our health. For years, I viewed eating as one of my favorite hobbies. I would eat first thing in the morning, all throughout the day, and as the last thing I did before going to bed. As I got older, my metabolism slowed down, but not my eating.

In November of 2013, I dedicated my body to the Lord and made a commitment to Him to live a healthier lifestyle, and I knew I had to start with nutrition. I started eating healthy food, finding some I liked, and even finding some that I really loved! I found out that if I ate the right kind of food in the right amount at the right times, I would never go hungry.

When someone asks you "for the hope that is in you" through your Imagine Not as Much journey, if you have committed your weight loss to God, you can confidently say that you will succeed because you have given it over to the Lord.

TAMMY'S TIDBITS

Since you have been eating healthier, I trust that you have also found a vegetable that you thought you didn't like but discovered you love. Share this new love with someone, and that can bring about a discussion about your story.

WEEK 12: DAY 4

Memory Verse: "But in your hearts regard Christ the Lord as holy, ready at any time to give a defense to anyone who asks you for a reason for the hope that is in you" (1 Peter 3:15).

Challenge: This week, share your story with someone who has not heard it.

Challenge Check-up: Have you found someone yet with whom to share your story? If not, pray earnestly that God will send someone in your path for the remainder of this week, so you can tell them of the good things God has done in your life, especially your relationship with the Lord Jesus Christ as Savior!

Focus: Benefits of Effective Time Management

NATHAN'S NOTIONS

With our focus today on the benefits of effective time management, we will spend time with the words in our memory verse: "ready at any time." As we think of readiness to give a defense to those who ask of the hope within our hearts, a few words will guide our thoughts: knowledge, affection, and courage.

The word *knowledge* reminds us that we must always stay aware of the people in our surroundings. We do not know where or when we will engage someone in a conversation; therefore, we need to stand ready at any time.

The second word, *affection*, reminds us that because we love people, we always want the very best for them. Our love and affection for the people we know will drive our desire to tell them what God has done, and continues to do, as we give our bodies to Him for His glory.

The third word, *courage*, reminds us that we can always trust the Lord's leadership when it comes to standing ready to give an answer of the hope that resides in our hearts. It takes courage to open up to someone and share with them that you struggle.

As we think about the benefits of effective time management, I want to stress the importance of setting specific goals for short-term success. This week, be "ready at any time" to tell someone your success story as you give your body to God for His glory!

TAMMY'S TIDBITS

Consolidate your story in writing as an effective way to share your story and manage your time. In this way, you can share your story with confidence. It does not have to be word for word but will give you a general idea of what to say.

WEEK 12: DAY 5

Memory Verse: "But in your hearts regard Christ the Lord as holy, ready at any time to give a defense to anyone who asks you for a reason for the hope that is in you" (1 Peter 3:15).

Challenge: This week, share your story with someone who has not heard it.

Focus: Physical Fitness

NATHAN'S NOTIONS

In our devotion time today, we will deal with the words "to give a defense to anyone who asks you." To "give a defense" in English translates one word in Greek, *apologian*.[40] As Peter uses the word, it serves two functions: a defense of the truth and for the good of the one asking. We should have the ability to give a reasonable explanation of why we do what we do so others can benefit. We need to make crystal clear that our motivation to lose weight springs out of our devotion to serve God.

In order to more effectively lose weight, one needs to add physical fitness to their daily routine. I engage in physical fitness to honor God with my body. We can also follow Peter's second reason for our *apologian* and share with them the benefit they could receive if they joined us. Losing weight comprises a hard fight against obesity that takes everything we have to gain the victory.

This week, prepare for your *apologian*. Prepare to give a defense of the things you do to lose weight and to keep it off. Prepare to stop the doubting of the naysayers by faithfully defending your decision to live a healthy life not only with your words, but also with your actions. Prepare to speak the truth in love, and prepare to do so in a way that might encourage someone to join you in your journey of Imagine Not as Much.

TAMMY'S TIDBITS

Just as we prepare to exercise, we should prepare to share. I recall the Scripture verse, Colossians 3:12b, which says, "Put on compassion, kindness, humility, gentleness, and patience." Another way to put this is to say "clothe yourselves." I know that as I get ready to exercise, I wear different clothes. In the same way, we should prepare ourselves for sharing. Share your story from your heart.

---

40 Joseph Henry Thayer, *A Greek-English Lexicon of the New Testament* (Edinburgh: T & T Clark, 1901), 65.

WEEK 12: DAY 6

Memory Verse: "But in your hearts regard Christ the Lord as holy, ready at any time to give a defense to anyone who asks you for a reason for the hope that is in you" (1 Peter 3:15).

Challenge: This week, share your story with someone who has not heard it.

Focus: Benefits of Friends

NATHAN'S NOTIONS

For today's devotion time, we will focus on the words that follow our memory verse from 1 Peter 3:16a: "Yet do this with gentleness and respect."

It does no good to offer an *apologian* in the wrong way. We should answer with gentleness and meekness toward the one asking to avoid pride or bitterness. We should answer in a humble spirit, with respect and fear, wanting anyone who asks of the hope we have to experience the same in their own lives. We should never take lightly the Divine nature of our journey. As we consider the truth of giving a defense of why we do things for God's glory, we should approach that task with a certain amount of respectful fear lest we injure our own souls by not speaking the truth, lest we injure the one who asks, and lest we injure God.

When we think about the awesome responsibility and weight upon our shoulders of answering those who ask of our hope, we can remember the benefits of friends. They will laugh, cry, or pray with us—whatever it takes to help us accomplish our goal. They will laugh at us when we make stupid mistakes, and they will cry with us when we suffer serious setbacks. Friends will pray with us for strength to continue each day and for us to keep going strong until we reach our goal! This week, invite your friends to help you practice gentleness and respect as you answer those who ask of the hope in your heart.

TAMMY'S TIDBITS

Our friends stick with us through thick and thin, through good and bad. I thank God for my friends. Each person stands unique in the sight of God, and so each person has a different story to tell. Your unique struggles can and will help someone else if you have the courage to share your story. Your story may encourage someone else in a way no one else's story can.

WEEK 12: DAY 7

Memory Verse: "But in your hearts regard Christ the Lord as holy, ready at any time to give a defense to anyone who asks you for a reason for the hope that is in you" (1 Peter 3:15).

Challenge: This week, share your story with someone who has not heard it.

Challenge Carry-over: Make a point to recognize when God brings somebody new into your sphere of influence, and share with them how you came to know the Lord Jesus Christ through a personal relationship with Him. Also, take time to share with them how you honor God with your body through *Imagine Not as Much*!

Focus: Motivational Fitness

NATHAN'S NOTIONS

In today's devotion time, we will consider again the benefits of following the advice in our memory verse: "But in your hearts regard Christ the Lord as holy." This will especially help us as we focus on motivational fitness. We can expect several benefits from setting apart the Messiah as Lord.

We can expect to allay any fear of what man may do to us. He stands alone as all-powerful and ever-present when we need a special touch of His hand. We can expect impure and unholy thoughts to diminish. The more we give our hearts and minds to the Lord, the less unholy and impure thoughts take root and infiltrate the rest of our bodies. We can expect unkindness, ill-opinion, and disrespect to disintegrate from our hearts. The Lord, Who lives in our hearts and controls our minds, loves every single person on this earth. We can expect patience when things do not go our way or when we experience bodily pain or distress in spirit. We sense the presence of God in the midst of pain, and we trust that God has a plan through what we must suffer.

Today, and for the rest of your life, "in your hearts regard Christ the Lord as holy," enjoying all the benefits that come from doing so.

TAMMY'S TIDBITS

I hope that you have shared your story this week. If so, please let us know; we would love to hear about it. If not, continue to pray for the opportunity. You will feel the presence of the Lord when you share your story with others. You may see great rejoicing because someone will have a closer relationship with the Lord, and He used you as an instrument in that process. You may also see great rejoicing because you obeyed, shared your story, and now have a closer relationship with the Lord. Great and wonderful things can and will happen!

CELEBRATION

When we lead this course at our church, we prepare to celebrate on week thirteen. We plan a healthy celebration potluck meal! We ask our Imaginators to bring a healthy dish, along with the recipe, for everyone to enjoy. We also ask them to invite a loved one, or someone they think might be interested in joining our group for the next session. We plan the menu during our week twelve session to make sure that we have enough healthy fruits and vegetables, starches, proteins, and desserts.

After we share the meal together, we each talk about what we have learned from participating in the program. We make plans to keep in contact until the next session. We share how our lives have changed since starting this weight loss journey and encourage each other to continue.

If you have picked up this book on your own and have not been part of group, how can you celebrate? Invite close family and friends to your house for a healthy meal or out to eat at your favorite restaurant for healthy foods—"Dutch treat," of course. Tell them you have changed your eating habits and how much better you feel. Ask for their support. If there is enough interest, you may want to start your own group! You will find as you lose weight and people begin to notice, that they will ask you how you did that.

WEEK 13: DAY 1

Memory Verse: "God also said, 'Look, I have given you every seed-bearing plant on the surface of the entire earth and every tree whose fruit contains seed. This will be food for you.'"

Challenge: This week, eat at least four to eight servings of fruits and vegetables every day.

Focus: Nutritional Fitness

NATHAN'S NOTIONS

In today's devotion, we want to spend some time on the amazing characteristics of food. In our memory verse, God says, "This will be food for you." God created food in all of its forms to sustain our daily living when used properly. But food entails much more than just sustenance; food has a power in and of itself.

At one time in history, people thrived in an agricultural society. Acquiring food entailed hard work and planning ahead to make sure you had enough to last through the winter. In our country, we live in a society where food comes easily and in excess. We can buy almost any food we need at the local store and prepare it at home in just a few minutes. We can satisfy almost every craving imaginable. We as a society no longer spend a great deal of time or energy in the production of food because we can find everything we need conveniently and quickly.

We as a society have lost the joy of eating simple, wholesome food as God created it. God gave us food to enjoy! He created the perfect fuel for our bodies by providing food for us in its natural state. When we eat the right kind of food in the right proportions and at the right times, we can rediscover a love affair with food that does not pose a danger to our bodies!

TAMMY'S TIDBITS

Every day this week, try to add a fruit or vegetable to your meal. I substituted celery for chips as one way to add vegetables and crunch with my lunch. In addition, I easily added lettuce and tomato to my sandwich.

WEEK 13: DAY 2

Memory Verse: "God also said, 'Look, I have given you every seed-bearing plant on the surface of the entire earth and every tree whose fruit contains seed. This will be food for you'" (Gen. 1:29).

Challenge: This week, eat at least four to eight servings of fruits and vegetables every day.

Focus: Benefits of Water

NATHAN'S NOTIONS

God not only has given us food, but He has also given us the most satisfying liquid on the planet to quench our thirst: wonderful water. Let's look at some simple reasons to choose water.

Water hydrates the body better than any other liquid with few or no side effects. I drank diet sodas, thinking that since they had no calories, they sufficed as a healthy alternative. I learned that the artificial sweeteners found in diet sodas triggered the production of insulin in my body, creating fat "storage"![41] Now that I primarily drink water, I no longer crave diet sodas.

Water does far more for us than we deserve. Some say water constitutes a minimalist approach to healthy living and should only serve as a choice of many other hydrating liquids. However, some research has shown that just a two-percent drop in water supply can trigger fuzzy short-term memory, trouble with basic math, and difficulty focusing on small print.[42]

We do not have to exert much effort to procure water for ourselves because God has supplied it abundantly. If we have access to a faucet or water fountain, we have access to water.

Water remains free from the temptation to excess. When we have had enough water, our bodies signal us to stop, and we do.

TAMMY'S TIDBITS

Recent research has indicated to drink at least sixty-four ounces a day up to half your body weight in ounces.[43] Have water constantly with you all throughout the day.

---

41 Batmanghelidj, 110-11.
42 Liz Neporent, *Fitness Walking for Dummies,* (Foster City: IDG Books Worldwide, Inc., 2000), 66.
43 Batmanghelidj, 135-36.

WEEK 13: DAY 3

Memory Verse: "God also said, 'Look, I have given you every seed-bearing plant on the surface of the entire earth and every tree whose fruit contains seed. This will be food for you'" (Gen. 1:29).

Challenge: This week, eat at least four to eight servings of fruits and vegetables every day.

Focus: Physical Fitness

NATHAN'S NOTIONS

As we focus on physical fitness during our devotional time today, we will consider the miracle of food as fuel for our bodies. God has given us the bounty of the land to consume to provide our bodies with the energy they need to function.

The kind of food and the amount of food we eat both determine what our bodies do with it. If we eat the right kinds of food in the right proportions and at the right times, we help our bodies function at optimum capacity. When we eat too much of the wrong kind of food, it takes one of two paths: either stored as fat or eliminated as waste. Our bodies can get rid of only so much waste a day; the excess it stores as fat.

God has provided all different kinds of food to help our bodies achieve optimum health. By following the Food Guide Pyramid along with the recommended caloric intake based on your weight loss goal, you will make sure that your body consumes the food it needs to accomplish physical fitness. By eating too little, you will not have the energy you need to exercise; and by eating too much, you will end up producing fat and waste.

TAMMY'S TIDBITS

It behooves us to find the time to engage in physical activity, no matter the season. Winter poses the greatest challenge for me to exercise. I find more excuses in this season to not stay physically active. I have never regretted exercising, but I almost always regret not exercising. Just go out, and do it.

WEEK 13: DAY 4

Memory Verse: "God also said, 'Look, I have given you every seed-bearing plant on the surface of the entire earth and every tree whose fruit contains seed. This will be food for you'" (Gen. 1:29).

Challenge: This week, eat at least four to eight servings of fruits and vegetables every day.

Challenge Check-up: How many days have you eaten at least four servings of fruits and vegetables this week? How many days have you eaten up to eight? If you have not succeeded, keep trying. Keep experimenting with different fruits and vegetables until you find several that you like and look forward to eating.

Focus: Benefits of Effective Time Management

NATHAN'S NOTIONS

In today's devotion time, we will expand our consideration of God's gift of food to incorporate His gift of the universe for us! God created the universe to show His love, to teach His truth, and to sustain our lives.

We can see the love of God in the extensiveness of the universe. The universe exists in such an astronomical enormity that it has proven difficult at best to assign a size to it. The universe teaches God's truth: that He exists, that He desires a relationship with us, and that He has a plan and purpose for each of us. The more we learn about the universe, the more we learn about the awesome nature of God. God's creation points to Him as Creator.

God created the universe to sustain our lives in perfect harmony with nature. He created air for us to breathe, water for us to drink, food for us to enjoy, and time for us in which to exist. God has provided time for each one of us. However, no one has unlimited time, so make the most of yours.

TAMMY'S TIDBITS

God knew exactly how many hours to put in a day. We want to stress the importance of sleep to our overall health. I have read multiple times that those who get at least seven hours of sleep lose weight faster than those who don't. Factor in a good night's sleep when you manage your time for overall good health.

WEEK 13: DAY 5

Memory Verse: "God also said, 'Look, I have given you every seed-bearing plant on the surface of the entire earth and every tree whose fruit contains seed. This will be food for you'" (Gen. 1:29).

Challenge: This week, eat at least four to eight servings of fruits and vegetables every day.

Focus: Motivational Fitness

NATHAN'S NOTIONS

In our focus on motivational fitness, we want to consider the reasons we should eat more fruits and vegetables. I want to make one thing perfectly clear: I love meat! However, I have discovered the joy of eating fruits and vegetables.

Nowhere in the text from Genesis chapter one does God say for man to eat meat. God gives him the charge to rule over the animals, but not to eat them. We have recorded in our memory verse the first food that God gave man to eat: fruits and vegetables. God does not give meat for man to eat until He speaks to Noah after the flood (Gen. 9:3).

God has provided fruits and vegetables in abundance, and we can attain them with relative ease from the store or our own gardens. If one puts their mind to it, they can find some that they enjoy. Sometimes, the way you prepare and cook vegetables makes all the difference in how they taste. You can grill, roast, boil, or steam vegetables. So, experiment this week. Stay motivated to eat the natural food God gave us to eat.

TAMMY'S TIDBITS

As Nathan stated, experimentation emerges as one way to motivate yourself to eat more fruits and vegetables. On your next trip to the grocery story, buy two or three fruits and vegetables that you do not know. Google healthy recipes that use these new fruits and veggies. This will give you something to look forward to, and you might find a new food that you enjoy!

WEEK 13: DAY 6

Memory Verse: "God also said, 'Look, I have given you every seed-bearing plant on the surface of the entire earth and every tree whose fruit contains seed. This will be food for you'" (Gen. 1:29).

Challenge: This week, eat at least four to eight servings of fruits and vegetables every day.

Focus: Benefits of Friends

NATHAN'S NOTIONS

In today's devotion time, we will look at the significance of the word *seed* in our memory verse. The Hebrew word *zera* refers to the unit of reproduction capable of developing into another such unit.[44] God designed fruits and vegetables to reproduce abundantly on the earth so that we humans would never lack a source of food.

Think about the phenomenal reproductive capability of seeds. One single plant of corn can produce six hundred seeds.[45] The power of multiplication becomes astronomical when one ponders the seed-bearing plants and fruits God has provided.

Our focus today centers on the benefits of friends. What if you became a seed? What if you remained faithful to your journey, lost weight, and became an inspiration for someone else? Maybe, just maybe, you will become the seed for the people who know you best to encourage them to live a healthy lifestyle for the glory of God. Through your obedience to the Lord and dedication to do all things for His glory, you just might emerge as the seed—not only of healthy living, but also as a germination of someone's spiritual health!

TAMMY'S TIDBITS

We can't wait for *you* to begin planting seeds and growing, too. One way to accomplish this comes by sharing with family and friends the healthy dishes that you have discovered.

---

44 H.W.F. Gesenius, *Gesenius' Hebrew-Chaldee Lexicon to the Old Testament* (Grand Rapids: Baker Book House, 1979), 253.
45 Dennis Elliott in a conversation with Nathan Whisnant.

WEEK 13: DAY 7

Memory Verse: "God also said, 'Look, I have given you every seed-bearing plant on the surface of the entire earth and every tree whose fruit contains seed. This will be food for you'" (Gen. 1:29).

Challenge: This week, eat at least four to eight servings of fruits and vegetables every day.

Challenge Carry-over: Hopefully, by now, you have discovered many fruits and vegetables that you enjoy. Keep eating them on a regular basis, making them a part of your daily food intake. You will feel healthier and act younger, and your body will say thank you!

Focus: Spiritual Fitness

NATHAN'S NOTIONS

In today's devotional time and focus on spiritual fitness, we will consider the words from our memory verse, "God also said, 'Look, I have given you.'" We can find food in such abundant supply, we may forget that what we eat comes from the gracious hand of God.

When we acknowledge that our food comes from God, we begin by offering Him thanks in prayer for the food He has provided. When we offer our humble prayers before God for the food He has given us, we truly understand the greatness of God's provision and the goodness of His mercy.

When we acknowledge that our food comes from the hand of God, we admit to Him our own beggary—meaning that without His bountiful supply, we would go without needed sustenance. Without God providing everything needed to produce food, we would have nothing to eat. He provides the earth's soil, the gentle rain, and the plentiful sunshine in just the right proportions to provide what we need. We develop spiritual fitness when we trust that God will always supply food for us.

TAMMY'S TIDBITS

First Thessalonians 5:18 says, "Give thanks in everything; for this is God's will for you in Christ Jesus." The apostle Paul encourages us to thank God in the good and in the bad. I find that when I thank God during the rough times, I grow closer to Him; and my faith grows. And the same remains true during good times, too. God provides, and we have trust and faith that He knows the best for us. Thank God, and praise Him for His majesty and all that He does!

CONCLUSION

Congratulations! If you have joined a group or taken this one week at a time, you may have lost over ten pounds by this point. Good for you! By now, you probably feel and look better.

Once again, thank you for taking the time to read this book. We believe you have invested valuable time to change your lifestyle for healthy living for a lifetime!

On this journey to pursue nutritional fitness, physical fitness, motivational fitness, and spiritual fitness, let's make John's statement about Jesus Christ ours—"He must increase, but I must decrease"—as we Imagine Not as Much.

"Now to him who is able to do above and beyond all that we ask or think according to the power that works in us—to him be glory in the church and in Christ Jesus to all generations, forever and ever. Amen" (Eph. 3:20-21).

APPENDIX A
SUGGESTED SERVINGS FROM EACH FOOD GROUP

The American Heart Association recommends eating a healthy diet full of fruits, vegetables, whole grains, and other nutritious foods. The table below shows the suggested number of servings from each food group based on a daily intake of 1,600 or 2,000 calories.

Food Type	1,600	2,000	Examples of One Serving
Grains	6 per day	6-8 per day	1 slice of bread 1 oz. dry cereal ½ cup cooked rice pasta or cereal

Food Type	1,600	2,000	Examples of One Serving
Vegetables	3-4 per day	4-5 per day	1 cup raw, leafy vegetables ½ cup cut up or raw cooked vegetables ½ cup vegetable juice

Food Type	1,600	2,000	Examples of One Serving
Fruits	4 per day	4-5 per day	1 medium fruit (the size of a baseball) ¼ cup dried fruit ½ cup fresh, frozen, or canned fruit ½ cup fruit juice

Food Type	1,600	2,000	Examples of One Serving
Dairy **Fat-free or low-fat**	2-3 per day	2-3 per day	1 cup milk 1 cup yogurt 1 ½ oz. cheese

Food Type	1,600	2,000	Examples of One Serving
Lean meats **Poultry, seafood** **Cooked weight**	3-6 per day	6 or less a day	3 oz. meat (size of a computer mouse) 3 oz. grilled fish (size of a checkbook)

Food Type	1,600	2,000	Examples of One Serving
Fats and oils	2 per day	2-3 per day	1 tsp. margarine 1 Tbsp. mayonnaise 1 tsp. vegetable oil 1 Tbsp. regular salad dressing 2 Tbsp. low-fat salad dressing

Food Type	1,600	2,000	Examples of One Serving
Nuts, seeds **Legumes**	3-4 per week	4-5 per week	1/3 cup or 1 ½ oz. nuts 3 Tbsp. peanut butter 2 Tbsp. or ½ oz. seeds ½ cup dry beans or peas

Food Type	1,600	2,000	Examples of One Serving
Sweets	0 per week	less than 5/week	1 Tbsp sugar 1 Tbsp jelly or jam ½ cup sorbet and ices 1 cup lemonade

APPENDIX B
HEALTHY FOODS

Calories per serving

FRUITS AND VEGETABLES

A

Apple,

Fuji	90 med.
Gala	79 med.
Golden Delicious	82 med.
Granny Smith	80 med.
Honey Crisp	80 med.
McIntosh	80 med.
Pink Lady	130 med.
Red Delicious	90 med.

Arrowroot	78 1 cup, sliced
Artichoke	76 1 large, raw
Asparagus	27 1 cup, raw
Avocado	289 1 fruit

B

Banana	105 med.

Beans,

Baked	239 1 cup
Black	227 1 cup
Chickpeas	286 1 cup
Kidney	215 1 cup
Lentils	226 1 cup
Pinto	245 1 cup
Refried	237 1 cup

Snap Green	44	1 cup
Beets, canned	49	1 cup
Blackberry	62	1 cup
Blueberry	83	1 cup
Bok Choy	50	½ head, raw
Broccoli	31	1 cup, raw
Brussels Sprouts	38	1 cup

C

Cabbage	22	1 cup, raw
Cantaloupe	60	1 cup
Capers	2	1 Tbsp.
Carambola (Star Fruit)	39	large
Carrot	25	1 med.
Cassava (Yuca)	330	1 cup, raw
Cauliflower	25	1 cup, raw
Celery	6	1 med. stalk
Chard	7	1 cup, raw
Cherries	74	1 cup
Chicory	41	1 cup raw
Chives	1	1 Tbsp.
Chrysanthemum, edible	6	1 cup, raw
Cilantro	10	50 g. raw
Coconut meat	159	45 g.
Coconut, sweet	70	2 Tbsp.
Collards	11	1 cup, raw
Corn	124	1 cup, raw
Cucumber	8	½ cup slices

D

Dandelion greens	25	1 cup, raw
Dill, dried	13	1 tsp.

E

Eggplant	21	1 cup, raw
Endive	4	½ cup, raw

F

Fennel, bulb	27 1 cup, sliced, raw
Fig, dried	47 uncooked

G

Garlic	4 1 clove
Gherkin	5 1 serving
Ginger	22 1 oz.
Grapes	62 1 cup
Guava	45 1 med.

H

Honeydew	64 1 cup
Horseradish, prep	7 1 Tbsp.
Huckleberry	10 1 oz.

J

Jicama	46 1 cup, raw

K

Kale	33 1 cup

L

Leek	50 1 med., raw
Lettuce	
Iceberg	7 1 cup
Mixed baby greens	15 2 cups
Romaine	15 2 cups
Spring Mix	19 3 cups

M

Macadamia	210 1 oz.
Mango	145 1 fruit
Mushroom	15 1 cup, raw
Portobello	22 1 cup, raw
Mustard	3 1 tsp.

N

Nectarine	62 1 med.

O

Okra	40 1 cup, raw
Onion	6 1 slice, med.
Oranges	62 1 fruit

P

Papaya	62 1 cup, raw
Paprika	6 1 tsp.
Parsley	22 1 cup
Parsnip	110 1 cup, sliced, raw
Passion Fruit	5 1 fruit
Peach	59 100 g.
Peas	117 1 cup, raw
Pear	96 1 med.
Pecan	98 10 pieces
Pepper	
Banana	9 1 small
Green	30 1 cup
Jalapeno	4 1 pepper
Sweet, red	46 1 cup
Yellow	50 1 large
Persimmon	118 1 fruit
Pimiento	25 100 g.
Pineapple	82 1 cup, chunks
Plantain	218 med.
Plum	20 1 fruit
Pomegranate	72 ½ cup
Potato	147 1 med., raw
Potato, sweet	100 130 g. fresh
Pumpkin	30 1 cup, raw

R

Radish	1 1 large
Raspberry	64 1 cup
Rhubarb	26 1 cup

Rutabaga	50	1 cup

S

Saffron	7	1 Tbsp.
Shallot	7	1 Tbsp.
Soybeans, edible	376	1 cup
Spinach	7	1 cup
Squash		
Butternut	63	1 cup
Spaghetti	20	¾ cup
Zucchini	20	1 cup
Yellow	49	1 cup
Strawberries	49	1 cup
Sweet basil	0	¼ tsp.
Swiss chard	7	1 cup

T

Tomatillo	11	1 med.
Tomato	16	1 small
Turnip	36	1 cup

W

Water Chestnut	36	4
Watercress	7	1 cup
Watermelon	46	1 cup

Y

Yams	177	1 cup

BEANS AND PEAS

Bean burgers	230	1 patty
Black beans	227	1 cup
Black-eyed peas	120	¾ cup
Falafel	57	1 patty
Garbanzo beans	286	1 cup
Kidney beans	215	1 cup

Lentils	226	1 cup
Lima beans	190	1 cup
Navy beans	296	1 cup
Pinto beans	245	1 cup
Soy beans	190	½ cup
Split peas	100	1 cup
White beans	110	½ cup

EGGS

Large	72

MEATS

Lean cuts of:

Beef	Cooked, Broiled	
Flank	165	3 oz.
Pot Roast, braised	282	3 oz.
Rib eye	174	3 oz.
Round	184	3 oz.
T-bone	168	3 oz.
Tenderloin	175	3 oz.
Top Sirloin	158	3 oz.
Veal, loin, roasted	364	1 piece

Lamb		
Lamb	184	3 oz.

Pork		
Ham, extra lean	30	1 slice
Pork chop	164	3 oz.

Game Meats		
Bison, top sirloin	145	3 oz.

Rabbit, stewed	32	1 oz.
Venison, roasted	46	1 oz.

Lean Ground Meats

Beef, cooked	145	3 oz.
Lamb, cooked	241	3 oz.
Pork, cooked	252	3 oz.

Organ Meats, Cooked

Beef liver	162	3 oz.
Chicken liver	234	1 cup

Lean luncheon or deli meats: varies per package

Poultry

Chicken, ground	160	4 oz., raw
Chicken, roasted	266	1 cup
Duck, roasted	281	1 cup
Goose, roasted	340	143 g.
Turkey, ground	170	4 oz., raw
Turkey, roasted	238	1 cup

NUTS AND SEEDS

Almonds	169	1 oz.
Cashews	162	1 oz.
Hazelnuts	200	¼ cup
Mixed nuts	168	1 oz.
Peanuts	166	1 oz.
Peanut butter	190	2 Tbsp.
Pecans	98	10 pieces
Pistachios	161	1 oz.
Pumpkin seeds	137	¼ cup
Sesame seeds	160	1 oz.

Sunflower seeds	165 1 oz.
Walnuts	200 ¼ cup

PROCESSED SOY PRODUCTS

Tofu	183 ½ cup, raw
Veggie burgers	114 1 burger

SEAFOOD

Canned fish:

Anchovies, drained	68 3 oz.
Clams, drained	126 3 oz.
Sardine, spring water	164 1 can
Tuna, drained	191 1 can

Fin-fish such as: Dry heat, Wild

Catfish	150 1 fillet
Cod, Atlantic	189 1 fillet
Cod, Pacific	95 1 fillet
Flounder	100 3 oz.
Haddock	168 1 fillet
Halibut	318 ½ fillet
Herring	290 1 fillet
Mackerel	231 1 fillet
Pollock, Atlantic	189 1 fillet
Pollock, Walleye	68 1 fillet
Salmon, Atlantic	280 ½ fillet
Sea Bass	125 1 fillet
Snapper	218 1 fillet
Swordfish	164 1 piece
Trout, rainbow	215 1 fillet
Tuna, yellow-fin	118 3 oz.

Shellfish:

Clams	168 1 cup, raw
Crab, blue	120 1 cup, cooked
Crayfish, wild	70 3 oz., cooked
Lobster, cooked	130 1 cup
Mussels, cooked	146 3 oz.
Octopus, cooked	139 3 oz.
Scallops, raw	26 2 large
Scallops, raw	26 5 small
Shrimp, cooked	101 3 oz.
Squid, raw	23 1 oz.

STARCHES

We should eat healthy starches, also known as carbohydrates, for a balanced diet. They produce lots of energy for the body. They contain calcium, iron, vitamin B, and fiber. Healthy starches can help reduce cholesterol levels, control blood glucose levels, and aid in weight loss. They include:

- Whole grains, such as whole wheat pasta, whole wheat bread, brown rice, oatmeal, and barley
- Starchy vegetables, such as corn, potatoes, squash, peas, and yams
- Beans, any variety

APPENDIX C
RECIPES

1.Grilled cheese sandwich with Light Savory Vegetable Barley soup

Top an open-faced, light English muffin with tomato slices, and sprinkle with shredded, low-fat mozzarella cheese or fat-free shredded cheese. Heat in oven until cheese melts. Heat soup according to directions. Servings vary.

2.Pita bread surprise with a salad

Preheat oven to 350 degrees. In a nonstick skillet, brown 93% fat-free ground beef with an onion in one tablespoon of extra virgin olive oil. Drain. Add taco mix and water according to directions on package, one cup of salsa, and one can of dark red kidney beans. Cook ten minutes. Place four whole wheat pita breads on a cookie sheet covered in aluminum foil treated with non-stick spray. Divide the meat mixture evenly on all four, and cover with an eight-ounce bag of shredded, low-fat mozzarella cheese or shredded fat-free cheese. Heat in the oven ten minutes. Add a salad for a side dish. Serves four.

3.Sirloin steak with baked potato and salad

Brown steak on a grill for ten minutes, or place on a grill. Add a baked potato and a salad as side dishes. Servings vary.

4.Shrimp stir-fry with brown rice

Stir-fry shrimp. Heat one tablespoon of extra virgin olive oil in a nonstick skillet over medium-high heat. Add garlic. Cook, stirring thirty to sixty seconds. Add shrimp in one layer. Cook three to five minutes per side (until shrimp is pink). Remove from pan. Add coleslaw mix, onions, and stir-fry veggies. Cook, stirring five to ten minutes until tender. Return shrimp to pan; top with teriyaki sauce; toss to heat through. Serve over brown rice. Servings vary.

5. Chicken tacos with brown rice and black beans

Heat a nonstick skillet with one tablespoon of extra virgin olive oil. Add one pound of chopped skinless, boneless chicken and an onion. Cook until all chicken is white; drain. Add taco mix and water according to directions on package and one cup of salsa. Make brown rice according to directions, and add one can of drained black beans. Heat whole wheat taco-size flour tortillas. Add chicken mixture; lettuce; tomato; low-fat, shredded mozzarella cheese or fat-free shredded cheese; and fat-free sour cream. Serves four.

6. Parmesan chicken with Brussel sprouts and wild rice

Sprinkle one pound of grilled skinless, boneless chicken breasts with seasoning salt. Cook on an indoor grill. Place them on a cookie sheet covered in aluminum foil treated with non-stick spray. Cover with one can of tomato sauce and an eight-ounce package of low-fat, shredded mozzarella cheese or fat-free, shredded cheese. Preheat oven to 350 degrees. Place Brussel sprouts in a gallon-size plastic bag, and coat with extra virgin olive oil, one teaspoon per person. Shake well. Spread on a cookie sheet covered with aluminum foil treated with non-stick spray. Salt and pepper to taste. Place in a preheated oven for fifteen minutes. Remove from oven. Flip over Brussel sprouts; salt and pepper to taste. Place back in oven for no more than fifteen more minutes, removing when Brussel sprouts begin to turn dark. When Brussel sprouts have been flipped and placed back in the oven, also place the Parmesan chicken in the oven. Make wild rice according to package directions as another side dish. Serves four.

7. Couscous chicken and vegetables with a salad

Sprinkle one pound of boneless, skinless chicken breast with seasoning salt. Cook on an indoor grill. Chop. Sauté four peppers and an onion with one tablespoon of extra virgin olive oil. Once vegetables are tender, add chicken and one can of tomato sauce, heating until sauce is warm. Prepare couscous according to package directions. Combine all ingredients together. Add a salad as a side dish. Serves four.

8. Spaghetti with a salad

Boil water. Add whole wheat spaghetti noodles. Brown ninety-three percent lean ground beef and an onion with one tablespoon of extra virgin olive oil in a nonstick skillet. Drain. Add spaghetti sauce of your choice. Heat until warm. Add a salad as a side dish. Serves four.

9. Pork chops with broccoli/cauliflower/onions and mashed potatoes

Cook pork chops on an indoor grill, adding seasoning to taste. Heat broccoli/cauliflower and onion with one tablespoon of extra virgin olive oil in a nonstick skillet. Cook mashed potatoes according to directions on package. Servings vary.

10. Loaded baked potato with Light Savory Vegetable Barley soup

Top a split baked potato with steamed broccoli and low-fat, shredded mozzarella cheese or fat-free, shredded cheese. Microwave until cheese begins to melt. Top with salsa and fat-free sour cream. Heat soup according to directions. Servings vary.

11. Turkey polish sausage/cabbage and onions with mashed potatoes and green beans

Heat turkey polish sausage and an onion in a large pot with one tablespoon of extra virgin olive oil. Add chopped cabbage. Continue to add cabbage. Cook until cabbage is tender, adding extra virgin olive oil as needed. Add green beans as a side dish, boiling them down after adding seasoning to taste and sugar or sugar substitute. Add mashed potatoes as a side dish. Serves four.

12. Lemon pepper chicken with oven-roasted vegetables and a rice dish

(For oven-roasted vegetables, make with a red onion, asparagus, four peppers, two squash, two zucchini, olive oil, salt and pepper). Sprinkle one pound of skinless, boneless chicken with lemon pepper seasoning. Make the chicken on an indoor grill. Preheat oven to 450 degrees. Cut up vegetables, and place in a glass baking dish that has been treated with cooking spray. Cover with three tablespoons of extra virgin olive oil. Salt and pepper to taste. Stir. Place dish in preheated oven for thirty minutes, stirring after ten minutes and stirring again before it is done. Prepare rice according to directions on package. Serves four.

13. Sirloin steak fajitas, brown rice with black beans

Make one pound of sirloin steaks on an indoor grill, seasoning to taste. Sauté four peppers and an onion in a nonstick skillet with one tablespoon of extra virgin olive oil. Add cooked steak, fajita mix, and water according to instructions on package. (Some fajita packages encourage marinating the steak before cooking; be sure to check the package you use.) Cook brown rice according to instructions, and add one can of black beans. Heat whole wheat taco-sized flour tortillas. Fill tortillas with steak mixture, lettuce, tomato, low-fat mozzarella shredded cheese or fat-free shredded cheese, and fat-free sour cream. Serves four.

14.Chicken teriyaki with brown rice, frozen bag of sugar snap pea stir-fry, and a salad

Make one pound of chopped chicken sprinkled with seasoning salt on an indoor grill. Heat bag of sugar snap pea stir-fry in a nonstick skillet according to directions with one table-spoon of extra virgin olive oil. Add grilled chicken and teriyaki sauce to taste. Simmer until sauce is warm. Cook brown rice according to directions on the package. On a plate, cover the brown rice with the chicken teriyaki mix. Add a salad as a side dish. Serves four.

15.Tuna patties with spinach and a baked potato

Heat one tablespoon of extra virgin olive oil in a non-stick skillet. Drain one can of tuna packed in water for each person. In a bowl, add to the drained tuna one beaten egg, half a package of whole wheat crackers crumbled (or one package of a fresh stack of whole wheat crackers crumbled), and mustard to taste. Mix well with hands. Form into a patty, and place carefully in heated skillet. Wait until edges start to turn brown; then carefully flip. Heat until done, when both sides have a rich, brown color. Heat spinach on stove top or microwave, add-ing vinegar and spices to taste as a side dish. Add a baked potato as a side dish. Servings vary.

16.Homemade pizza with a salad

Start with whole wheat pizza dough. Cook according to instructions. Top with pizza sauce and vegetables of your choice. Use ninety-three percent lean ground beef or turkey pep-peroni for meat. Cover with low-fat, shredded mozzarella cheese or fat-free, shredded cheese; and bake according to instructions. Add a salad as a side dish. Servings vary.

17.Bow-tie (or different variety) pasta with chicken and a salad

Sprinkle one pound of boneless, skinless chicken with seasoning salt, and make on a George Foreman or a grill. Sauté roasted, chopped tomatoes, four peppers, onion, two squash, and two zucchinis in a nonstick skillet with one tablespoon of extra virgin olive oil. Add chicken when it is done. Cook whole wheat pasta according to package instructions. Combine cooked whole wheat pasta with chicken and vegetables. Sprinkle with Italian herbs and one 8-ounce package of fat-free, shredded mozzarella cheese or fat-free, shredded cheese. Mix well Serves four.

18. Barbecue chicken with asparagus and wild rice

Sprinkle one pound of boneless, skinless chicken with seasoning salt, and make on an indoor grill. Coat with barbecue sauce to taste. Preheat oven to 350 degrees. Cover a cookie sheet with aluminum foil treated with nonstick spray. Keep asparagus whole; place in a gallon plastic bag with one teaspoon extra virgin olive oil per person served. Shake well. Spread evenly on prepared cookie sheet. Add salt and pepper to taste. Bake for fifteen minutes. Take out; flip; and add more salt and pepper to taste. Cook no longer than fifteen more minutes, removing when the asparagus begins to turn dark. Cook wild rice according to directions on package as another side dish. Serves four.

19. Grillers or Brats/sautéed green peppers and onions with macaroni and cheese and a salad

Make grillers/Brats in a nonstick skillet with one tablespoon of extra virgin olive oil or grill until done to taste. Sauté green peppers and onion in a skillet with one tablespoon extra virgin olive oil until tender and turning dark. Top with condiments of your choice. If buns are used, be sure to use whole wheat. Make macaroni and cheese and a salad as side dishes. Servings vary.

20. Chicken enchiladas with brown rice and black beans and a salad

Sprinkle one pound of skinless boneless chicken with seasoning salt and chop. Cook chicken and onion in a nonstick skillet with one tablespoon of extra virgin olive oil. When chicken is white, drain. Add taco mix and water according to package instructions with one cup of salsa. Preheat oven to 350 degrees. Divide chicken mixture into eight equal parts, and place in eight taco-sized whole wheat flour tortillas. Place these in a glass baking dish that has been treated with non-stick cooking spray. Cover items in the dish with one can of enchilada sauce and an eight-ounce package of low-fat, shredded mozzarella cheese or fat-free, shredded cheese. Upon plating, cover two enchiladas with fat-free sour cream. Make brown rice according to instructions, and add one can of black beans as a side dish. Add a salad as another side dish. Serves four.

21. Grilled ham with green beans and mashed potatoes

Make grilled ham on a George Foreman or a grill. Boil down green beans, adding seasoning to taste and sugar or a sugar substitute. Make mashed potatoes according to directions. Servings vary.

22. Seasoned salt chicken with squash/zucchini/onions and Rice-a-Roni

Sprinkle chicken with seasoning salt, and cook on a George Foreman or a grill. Sauté chopped squash, zucchini, and onion in a nonstick skillet with one tablespoon of extra virgin olive oil. Prepare Rice-a-Roni according to package directions. Servings vary.

23. Flounder with couscous and a salad

Brush both sides of flounder with extra virgin olive oil, and sprinkle one side with lemon pepper seasoning. Cook on an indoor grill or a nonstick skillet. Make couscous according to package directions, and add a salad as side dishes. Servings vary.

24. Breakfast with turkey sausage patties, hash brown potatoes/onions, eggs, and whole wheat toast with jelly

Make frozen potatoes according to package directions in a nonstick skillet with one tablespoon of extra virgin olive oil, adding a chopped onion. Prepare turkey sausage in a skillet according to package directions with one tablespoon of olive oil. Make two eggs to taste and two pieces of whole wheat toast with one tablespoon of jelly per slice. Servings vary.

25. Hamburgers with French fries and a salad

Preheat oven to 450 degrees. Make whole potatoes (one medium to large size per person) into French fries, and place in a gallon-size plastic bag. Cover with one teaspoon extra virgin olive oil per person. Shake well. Cover a cookie sheet with aluminum foil treated with nonstick cooking spray. Place French fries on prepared cookie sheet in one even layer. Salt and pepper to taste. Place in the oven for fifteen minutes. Remove; flip fries; salt and pepper to taste again; and place back in the oven for no longer than fifteen minutes, removing the fries when they are golden brown. Use one pound of ninety-three percent fat-free ground beef, and form into hamburger patties. Season to taste. Make on an indoor grill. Top with fat-free, sliced cheese on a whole wheat bun or whole wheat bread, or no bread if preferred. Use condiments to taste. Add a salad as a side dish. Servings vary.

BIBLIOGRAPHY

Aland, Kurt, Matthew Black, Carlom Martini, Bruce M. Metzger, and Allen Wikgren, eds., *The Greek New Testament/Dictionary Third Edition* Corrected. Munster/Westphalia: United Bible Societies, 1966-1983.

Batmanghelidj, Fereydoon. M.D. *Your Body's Many Cries for Water: You're Not Sick; You're Thirsty. Don't Treat Thirst with Medications.* Falls Church: Global Health Solutions, Inc., 2008.

Bushman, Barbara, Editor. *American College of Sports Medicine Complete Guide to Fitness & Health: Physical Activity and Nutrition Guidelines for Every Age.* Champaign: Human Kinetics, 2011.

Cruise, Jorge. *8 Minutes in the Morning.* New York: HarperCollins Publishers, 2003.

Cruise, Jorge. *8 Minutes in the Morning for Real Shapes Real Sizes.* New York: Rodale, 2003.

Ferguson, James M, M.D., and Cassandra Ferguson. *Habits Not Diets: The Secret to Lifetime Weight Control.* Boulder: Bull Publishing Company, 2003.

Fuhrman, Joel, M.D. *The End of Dieting: How to Live for Life.* New York: HarperCollins Publishers, 2014.

Gesenius, H.W.F., *Gesenius' Hebrew-Chaldee Lexicon to the Old Testament.* Grand Rapids: Baker Book House, 1979.

Green, Jay P., Sr. ed., *The Interlinear Hebrew/Greek-English Bible.* 4 vols. Lafayette: Associated Publishers & Authors, Inc., 1976-1984.

Greene, Bob. *Bob Greene's Total Body Makeover: An Accelerated Program of Exercise for Maximum Results in Minimum Time.* New York: Simon & Schuster Paperbacks, 2005.

Kittel,G, and G. Friedrich, eds. *Theological Dictionary of the New Testament.* Translated by G.W. Bromiley. 10 vols. Grand Rapids: Eerdmans, 1964-1976.

Lotz, Anne Graham. "God of the Impossible on 1 Peter 5:7." Daily Light for Daily Living Radio. Raleigh: AnGel Ministries. April 6, 2017.

Neporent, Liz, M.A. *Fitness Walking for Dummies.* Foster City: IDG Books Worldwide, Inc., 2000.

Reinhard, Tonia, MS, RD. *Super Foods: The Healthiest Foods on the Planet.* Buffalo: Firefly Books, 2014.

Reynolds, Steve. *Bod4God: The Four Keys to Weight Loss.* Ventura: Regal from Gospel Light, 2009.

Snyderman, Nancy L., M.D. *Diet Myths That Keep Us Fat and the 101 Truths that Will Save Your Waistline—and Maybe Even Your Life.* New York: Crown Publishers, 2009.

Thayer, Joseph Henry. *A Greek-English Lexicon of the New Testament.* Edinburgh: T & T Clark, 1901.

Tumminello, Nick. *Strength Training for Fat Loss: Lose Fat, Develop Lean Muscle, Improve Health, Feel Great.* Champaign: Human Kinetics, 2014.

Warner, Jackie. *This Is Why You're Fat (And How to Get Thin Forever): Eat More, Cheat More, Lose More—and Keep the Weight Off.* New York: Wellness Central, 2010.

Weight Watchers International, Inc. *Weightwatchers What to Cook Now: 300 Recipes for Every Kitchen.* New York: St. Martin's Griffin, 2014.

Wright, Vonda, and Ruth Winter. *Fitness After 40: How to Stay Strong at Any Age.* New York: Amacom Books, 2009.

Zinczenko, David, and Matt Goulding. *Cook This Not That! The No-Diet Weight Loss Solution.* New York: Rodale, 2010.

Zinczenko, David, and Matt Goulding. *Eat This Not That! Restaurant Guide: The No-Diet Weight Loss Solution.* New York: Rodale, 2010.

For more information about

Nathan and Tammy Whisnant
and
Imagine Not As Much
please connect at:

www.nathanandtammyw.com
Nathanandtammyw@gmail.com

For more information about
AMBASSADOR INTERNATIONAL
please connect at:

www.ambassador-international.com
@AmbassadorIntl
www.facebook.com/AmbassadorIntl

If you enjoyed this book, please consider leaving us a review on
Amazon, Goodreads, or our website.

More from Ambassador International

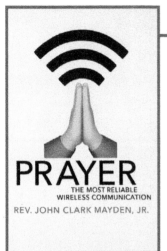

In today's world of instant communication, any problems with cellular service or Wi-Fi access can be a major disruption to one's day. But there is one kind of communication that is always reliable and never disrupts: prayer.

Prayer: The Most Reliable Wireless Communication
by Rev. John Clark Mayden, Jr.

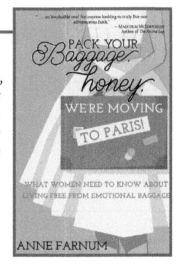

Everyone has baggage!

We all have something that keeps us from living fully for the Lord, but Christ wants us to give our baggage to Him so we can follow Him freely. In *Pack Your Baggage, Honey, We're Moving to Paris!* Anne Farnum explores the different kinds of baggage we carry. She also focuses on the baggage that King Saul hid behind and compares it to that which David left behind to run toward the giant.

Pack Your Baggage, Honey, We're Moving to Paris!

by Anne Farnum

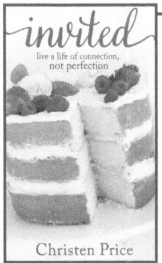

With kindness, honesty, and Biblical truth, author Christen Price encourages readers to overcome the hurdles of perfection by finding balance instead of breaking down, receiving others in love by releasing all anxieties to God and rejoicing in the moments worth celebrating, and discovering that the antidote to perfection is embracing the beauty of imperfection and presenting not only yourself, but your home, in an artful way so you can give and receive joy.

Invited

by Christen Price